Hearing a Different Voice

Spiritual Intervention for the Autistic Spectrum Disorder, *ADHD/ADD and Learning Disabilities.*

Consuelo Cassotti B.S.

Edited by Tehya Whitehawk
Copyright © 2013 Cover Image by Consuelo Cassotti
"I AM the Deep Truth" acrylic painting

Copyright © 2013 by Consuelo Cassotti

Note from the author:
All the children's, teenagers' and parents' names have been changed with the purpose to protect their privacy.

ISBN: 1-4810-9871-3
ISBN-13: 9781481098717

dedication: This book is written with love and the desire to show a new way to look at energy work. I would like to thank all of my friends who have supported me in this endeavor, but in particular Julie Snoeberger, Tehya Whitehawk, Phyllis Pacifico, Echo Wright and Gloria De Giuseppe. Thanks to each of the children and their parents who, with their trust, have given me the opportunity to better learn and understand my work. Thanks also to my husband, Giovanni, and my family.

Contents

"We are all connected. Sooner or later, if you are open to listening you are going to figure out the reason why we have met".

- Consuelo Cassotti

introduction: As an empathic and intuitive person, I have always had a natural predisposition to feeling and hearing that differs from most. My move from Italy to the United States prompted me to look ever deeper within myself, bringing to light previously unrealized skills. I also feel very blessed, having found incredible spiritual friends in a new country, whom I refer to as my "Galactic Family." They have helped me to better understand my path and follow it. This is an incredible journey... a great occasion to connect through heart, and souls that seek awakening and the ability to follow their own path with harmony and joy. We are all connected in many ways. I discover that each time I give a session. I am able to speak "soul to soul" with the client. I can shift multi-dimensionally, and see other Light Beings working on the client as well. In this same way, I can easily give a long distance session to someone I've never met, or be the voice of those who cannot speak due to physical or emotional challenges.

My Typical Session

- Throughout the course of a session I work with different teams of Spiritual Guides and Angels, some related to the client or myself, and others as technical teams who arrive only for specific work during the session. For this reason, I will use the plural "we" or "they" during the session. This is because most of the time I don't physically touch the client, but rather I describe and explain their energetic work. Sometimes I participate in the session, helping the Lightworkers. Other times I just hold the "portal" and observe their work. In any case, I can reach the mind/soul of the person on the table, and as an empathic/facilitator I feel their emotions and see memories from this life or past lives.

- I cannot predict what is going to happen. Every session is different and very specific to the "real needs/priorities" of that particular client.

- One very interesting thing I have noticed is "wings" on people! I have learned that this is due to angelic encoding in the DNA. In some way, everyone is encoded with angelic energy. Whether one believes we were angels in another lifetime and it is part of our genetic heritage, or some other explanation, the way that clients reveal their wings to me gives me some metaphoric information about the person.

. I should emphasize here, that the conversation with the client is not a vocal one, but it is a "mind to mind" or "soul to soul" conversation between the client and myself. I can pick up sentences, images, and feelings during the session. The more open a client is, and the deeper he or she is willing to go, the greater my access to information.

. There are sections of the text where I have used the term *regular conversation*, and in that case I am referring to the client using his/her own natural voice.

Chapter 1
"The compassionate soul who needed to recognize all his parts"

When I was in Italy teaching some classes and visiting with my family, my dear friend Echo emailed me the phone number of a woman named Julie, who lived very close to me. Echo believed that she would be a good contact, and that it could possibly turn into a good friendship for the both of us. After my trip to Italy, I finally had occasion to meet Julie.

Immediately I felt that we were friends, with many shared past lives. I also had the impression that I could be very open with her, without any regrets afterward. In our first conversation, Julie told me that 11 years earlier her life had changed completely when her son JJ was diagnosed with Autism. When JJ was 2 years old they had to move to another State. Julie thought it would be better for JJ to receive all of his vaccinations before moving, as she was not sure if she could find a good pediatrician so soon in a new state. Unfortunately, without blinking an eye, JJ's pediatrician agreed.

JJ received five different shots in 2 days. After several days, he became very ill. He stopped speaking, his personality changed, and he had a loss of coordination. Everything about him changed. His lack of balance progressed to the point that he was a danger to himself. He had to wear a helmet for protection, as he took up the practice of banging his head against the wall.

JJ was diagnosed as Autistic, and several doctors told Julie that he would never recover. When she told them that she planned to help her son reach his full potential, they said that she was depressed and in denial. They suggested she take some medications and face the truth. Luckily, she decided to be more proactive instead!

This was a big wake up call for Julie. She decided not to go on medication, but instead sought to discover another solution, without the advice of "traditional doctors". She soon realized how intolerant and allergic JJ was becoming to many foods. After some research she started using only organic food. She prepared only fresh veggies, no more GMO and white flours. The more attention she paid to JJ's diet, the more she noticed improvements in JJ. Julie reached the point where she was always at home with JJ, isolated. She focused on using this time to find the best way to help her son. With better nutrition, supplements, and improved recipes...the whole family's diet changed!

Along with diet, Julie began to explore the holistic side of treatment including alternative therapies, energy work, and shamanistic techniques. Other parents of autistic children disagreed with her choices. Some felt that it was outside the Christian path, and therefore unacceptable. Julie believed that God is everywhere, and not bound by any one religion. Furthermore, she felt that God is in any spiritual person that works with an open heart, for the highest good of the soul. Julie's goal was to recover her son with harmony and love, and she was determined to reach that goal.

It was amazing, yet heartbreaking to hear how alone she felt. Julie had to learn to stand up for herself, and for her son. This was particularly difficult, as it would have been so easy to follow the "socially acceptable" path of medications and labeling! She shared with me the insight that she gained from her experience. Julie realized that what happened to JJ was meant to be. Her whole family's life changed. Of course it wasn't so simple, she often felt depressed, even suicidal at times. Her life was turned completely upside down, but little by little, piece by piece, anytime that she or JJ had energy work or shamanistic work done, things improved. She realized that she was on the right track. After years of great work with naturopathic doctors, Bodytalk, energy work and good food, JJ was experiencing good results.

ॐॐ

First session (January)

After we met, Julie decided to bring JJ to me for a session. At the time he was thirteen years old. When he arrived he seemed very restless, always fidgeting, walking around or moving his leg when he was seated. His speech was rapid and it was difficult for him to make direct eye contact. Julie assured me that he was accustomed to being on a massage table, and once he took his place on the table my session started.

I start the session. First we work on his nervous system, particularly the lower extremities, his legs and hips. I observe them working on his skin. They explain to me that his body is growing

3

and needs more help. I can see and feel the difficulty of his joints, as they are stretching and adapting to the change. His mind moves quickly, and it looks as though he has a hard time stopping it, or like he never does. His mind is full of thoughts. I can see memories, information, faces...it looks like "garbage". It is time to clean it, like a computer that needs to be rebooted. The Light Beings and I work on helping him to clear away some thoughts, old stuff that he didn't need any more.

They are suggesting me to explain to JJ that he doesn't need to use his old way of thinking (the way he thought when he was autistic), but that he can "switch" and begin to have a new way to think and act now. His autistic/nervous/obsessive pattern is part of the past. Now that JJ is growing up he can no longer relate to his old way of thinking.

We help him to release some anxiety and tension that he had been carrying around for some time. He has everything inside, all the knowledge he requires. His soul knows his mission. He doesn't need to fear the future, for he is past the hardest part of his life. Now it will be easier. The fact the he can feel so deeply and is more sensitive, gives him the impression that he is different from the other teenagers, but he needs to see this as something helpful. This will allow him to become the man he will be in the future.

The Future Self shows up. I see JJ as an 18/19 year old, well built body, smiling and confident. He says that he will be a creative technician, for a green environment... I believe that he is talking about a future specialized occupation. I have a hard time understanding exactly what he will do.

He explains that he chose this family. He wanted to be part of this family, because they will support him in this path.

My Spirit Guides tell me: "The hardest part of his life is done. All of this was necessary for him; he will use his life experience for his future mission/job.

His soul says that he missed his original home, but mostly because he had a difficult time fitting in with this society. He needs a little more time and help to realize how much he can do here".

JJ explains to me, that he can be happy because he feels loved. I can see that he is guided, and he seems also very confident about what he wants to be in the future. He has a mission and he is here to achieve it.

Because he has a hard time sleeping well, at the end of the session my Spirit Guides advise me to tell Julie to "massage his feet, and have him bathe in the evening. This will help to relax his nervous system. The session is over, I thank everybody ... "

I asked Julie to set up a session every 3-4 weeks (21 to 30 days). When we work with these children to change the old behaviors, it is necessary to have regular sessions in order to reinforce the new behaviors. Julie was happy to hear that JJ had put the old behaviors behind him. Some days later, she began to notice that JJ was more focused and calm. I was happy to see JJ improve in such a short time.

The fact that JJ was eating the right food, a diet without sugar, white flour, fast food and fried food, was very helpful. In fact, many times my Spirit Guides have told me to tell the parents of some children that I work with "More water!" or "Not so much sugar!" Other times, I can smell fried chicken or "French fries" during the session, particularly when we work on releasing toxins from the body.

Consuelo Cassotti B.S.

A healthy diet is an important aspect of health for everyone, but with ADD/ADHD and Spectrum Disorder children it is mandatory. My observation is that when these children are eating processed food and too much sugar, the liver becomes very busy, and needs a lot of energy from the body in order to filter and process the food. Because most of these children have an overactive mind, the body is already struggling to send a huge amount of energy to the brain. In the meantime, it must continue to help the other parts of the body to function regularly. If there is not enough energy in the body to handle everything, then we begin to see some imbalances and a lack of coordination. Speech is the first thing that is compromised.

When Julie and I spoke about this aspect, she shared with me an incredible experience that supports this theory. She said that just a week ago, she was advising a parent of a three years old autistic child to change his son's diet. A week after they changed his diet, the father phoned Julie to tell her the great news: for the first time, the little boy was starting to talk!

I have the impression that one of the reasons why there are more autistic children in the USA, is also because a lot of Americans have stopped cooking for themselves, and use only processed food. After Julie and I shared our experiences, we agreed that the best way to help these children is to apply these points:
-   Less medications
-   Energy work
-   Proper diet
-   Involve the whole family in the energy work

Again, we are all connected. The more we clear ourselves, and become aware of one another's energy, the easier it becomes for these children to be more balanced and happy. Your child can be absorbing emotions and stress as a natural healer or empathic. He/She may also have some past life issues. Your child may be absorbing your emotions, your sense of guilt, your anxiety and more. If you begin working on your issues, you can help both yourself and your child to be less affected by them, as well as any close relatives or the environment.

Julie's session (February):

Julie decided to have a session. She wanted to see if a connection between her and JJ would show up during the session, or any other important information that would help her to better understand her path with JJ. (She allowed me to describe her full session).

The session starts. I see a taller light being with very long hands working on her heart chakra, front and back. At the same time, she is receiving a lot of information through her crown chakra, which is wide open. She was downloading information. Other beings are working at her feet; they have an earthy energy, like young gnomes. They are also working on her skeleton, because it is time to change the structure of her body. It is about transformation. They work on her neck. They say that it is important to change the way that her body is supporting her head. It isn't about structure/posture, but related to an energetic connection. This change will cause her to be more connected. The occipitals are an important place for them to work. They work in the back of the head (the medulla) called "the chamber of God." In Italy it is called "The mouth of God."

They work on the spine and sacrum to help the body be more balanced. Julie reports feeling encircled by numerous light beings. Someone else is again working on her heart chakra. I observe her heart chakra, and it looks like a little tornado is inside the chakra. The being said that his work on Julie was to create an expansion of her heart. My Spirit Guide says regarding Julie: "You are the kind of person who is very connected to the Earth. You are deeply connected to this planet. You can feel the vibration. You can feel the movements of nature. This is the reason why these little people were on your feet. They were the link to the Earth, and they are connected to you too."

Another being with blonde hair, full of compassion and love, stands close to her at the top of her head. He touches his forehead to Julie's forehead. My Spirit Guide explains that this is a way to create a connection. I do not understand if this being is female or male, but I heard the name Aiael (or Aiel) ... Master Aiael. He says: "I am a master and I will support your intuitive part. Be nice to yourself, don't push yourself too much!" I ask if they have a message for Julie. They answer: "There is something or someone in Mount Shasta for you." It could be related to the Violet Flame, because I saw violet color.

The session continues. Now a woman from North Africa, like the nomadic Tuareg people, shows up. She begins painting a tattoo on Julie's legs with henna. She draws sacred geometries from her knees to her feet. This ceremony is related to the creation of a strong connection with the planet Earth.

They cover her entire body with an electric blue jelly that helps to change the body to the new vibration. They explain to me that this jelly is made mostly of water, because human cells are full of water. Raising the vibration of the body will be easily accomplished through the use of this jelly. Suddenly Julie becomes very emotional. They said to tell her to let go, and that this is part of something that she was asking for. The beings bless Julie, and thank her for letting it happen. They said: "You are very blessed, and because of this you are doing fine." They then said: "Julie, you are connected to Mt. Shasta from now on. If you go there with your heart open, you will receive what it is that you need."

Before the session finished, an Ethiopian woman shows up. She wears numerous ring necklaces on her long neck. She is one of Julie's spirit guides; she is Julie's connection to Africa. She explains that Julie has a past life in Africa as a medicine woman. Julie admits that she has always been curious about herbs and their properties.

We are at the end of the session. Everyone opens their arms and puts their hands on the top of her body, singing a particular sound. The one that was holding her heart earlier showed him-self. He looked like the fictional Vulcan. His ears are pointed and he has long fingers and arms. He is a very sweet guy.

The session is over. I thank everyone.

After her session Julie left, she was very happy and tired at the same time; she felt that she must go home and rest.

After some minutes, Julie called me and requested an appointment for her husband. JJ's father had been laid off from his company for some months, and this was affecting everybody.

Consuelo Cassotti B.S.

JJ's father's session

I am reporting only some brief parts that can help to understand the relationship between JJ and his family.

During the session I could feel his tension and the sense of responsibility for his family. He was really under a lot of stress. He used to have an important role in the company. His soul explained to me that he had created this situation, he was traveling a lot and he was starting to lose any connection with his wife and children. He was close to losing them forever. This was the last chance for him to re-connect before it was too late. He was very open to letting go of the tension and worries that he had carried for months. I saw his connection with his entire family during the session, as a past life memory with he and JJ as medieval warriors. My Spirit Guides asked me to inform him that he will be fine in a few months. They were very positive about his situation...

After the session we had a discussion about this. He admitted that he was taking his children to their school activities during the day, for the first time in his life, and that he enjoyed being more involved in their lives. He was feeling more recharged and relaxed. He felt as though a big, heavy weight was lifted from his shoulders.

The day after, Julie informed me that she noticed not only her husband be more relaxed and present; also JJ was positively affected by his father's session.

ॐ∾ॐ

Second session (February)

JJ was more focused, but in the last days Julie noticed that he was less grounded and present. The session would be a good help for him.

Immediately, as I am opening the session, they align all the chakras.

They say that it is necessary to energetically update all organs, because they need a higher vibration. JJ's soul said that he has a hard time relaxing completely and deeply. JJ feels stress from school.

His soul also expresses the desire to change, but one part of him (the actual personality) is afraid to lose the reference points. He has a hard time exchanging old habits for something new that he doesn't really know well. He expresses that one of the reasons why he has a hard time is because he is worried about the Void, the Space. To be in the Void without reference points, makes him feel as though he doesn't have any control. I feel that it is about letting go of the control, as his mind never stops...it is always spinning. We work to create more peace in his mind; we help him to be more calm and focused. I see in his mind like an infinity symbol, that goes very fast. We slow down this movement.

At the end of the session I begin to see water. I understand the connection to water and JJ is calmer and more relaxed. The water helps to relax the nervous system, to allow one to calm down more easily. The session is over. I thank everyone.

I advise Julie to have JJ bathe before going to sleep instead that take a shower, as the water can help him to relax. She said that he loved to take both showers and baths, probably for the same reason that I perceived.

Consuelo Cassotti B.S.

Julie's feed back by email, the day after:

"After the session we drove home. JJ fell asleep in the car and when we arrived at home, he was calm and tired. The next morning his face looked better, and he was more focused. His speech and movements confirmed this, as he was calmer and more coordinated".

రొళ

Third session (given by distance, March)

When I was in Italy, I gave long distance sessions to JJ and his parents. It was amazing to see how many positive changes Julie noticed in JJ, just after receiving a session from me.

It was time to give another session to JJ, which I did some days after his parents' session.

I need to clarify that this session was more like a "maintenance session."

I call it a maintenance session, as during the session I don't receive particular information, but we take care of the "regular stuff." Just like with a car: we change the oil, rotate the tires, and add some gasoline. Normally, it doesn't seem that we go very deep. *I have the impression that it is a session where we support the changes from the session before, as it sometimes takes time and assistance to integrate them.*

We begin to clear his thoughts, slow down his mind. We take care of the nervous system and help him to relax. We check all the body's parts and we change them energetically where necessary. We ground and balance him. We work also on any allergies related to the season, and his sinuses. He looks more balanced and has a good flow of energy. He doesn't need to go too deep.

We reinforce the belief systems that we worked with in other sessions. He knows that he can do anything he wants!

The session is over. I thank everyone.

My Spirit Guides explain to me that another reason why JJ has needed a light session is because I gave a prior session to his parents, just some days before. It is about connection. Family members are connected to each other emotionally and spiritually, not just physically. Because of this, sensitive children like autistics, easily absorb emotions and tensions from their family members.

Fourth session (April)

Before I began the session, Julie said that JJ would like to be more brawny and relaxed; he still has a hard time relaxing deeply. She also asked me to help integrate his ability to do better in math. I set these requests as intentions; I asked for his higher good to work on them.

Immediately upon beginning the session, I feel that JJ needs to be cleared of toxins, thoughts, emotions, and ideas...anything that cannot be released without energy work. His mind is always running so fast and this time is no different. We work to slow down and balance the mind. I ask my beings to increase his ability to do better in math, and they do it immediately. They start working at his head, on the crown chakra or third eye. They connect various points of energy in different parts of JJ's brain. It is taking some minutes...

We work on the spine to reach the Nervous System. Through the spine it is possible to reach all the nerves in the body, and the body parts connected to the nerves. The light beings work by focusing on specific points. I ask to help him acquire a well-built musculature. I send an image to JJ of himself with well built muscles, and a harmonious physique.

A Fairy arrives during the session. She wants to connect with him, and she knows JJ from other dimensions/life times. She explains that JJ is connected to her Kingdom and how he was a part of them in another period. Immediately I see a picture of him happy, surrounded by female and male fairies that welcome him home. Probably because of this Fairy connection, I feel a lighter energy in the room.

I also have the impression that JJ is releasing all the heaviness that he had when he arrived. The session was lighter and very focused on the specific priorities. The session is over. I thank everybody.

Because Julie and I have noticed great improvements in JJ, I have decided at this time to wait 5 to 6 weeks between sessions. His grades improved and he was more calm and focused.

అ౼ఌ

Fifth Session (end of May)
I immediately noticed that JJ was in need of a "battery recharge", but I did not want it to push him into a hyperactive state. The amount of stress from school was huge.

We began the session by clearing away any tiredness and thoughts from his mind and body. He falls asleep. I reinforce his Positive Future Self and remind him that he can be whomever he wants. We spend some moments in this conversation and he is lis-

tening. We work at this physical body, we recharge all his cells and help him to be more grounded. I receive no particular information, but I notice that as we work, we spend less time on his brain and his nervous system. I feel that it is because he is doing better. Everything seams to be lighter, JJ looks more balanced and very receptive for every thing we are doing. It becomes easy to give him the session. Half an hour is passed, the session is over. I thank everyone.

Early in June, Julie called me. She explained to me how hard she has always tried to push JJ to go to summer camp. She had always hoped that he would decide to go, because she felt that it would help JJ to build more confidence.

This summer, she brought up the conversation with JJ about summer camp, and like every other year, she anticipated the same reaction. This time however, JJ answered "Ok mom, but only if you let me choose the right camp for me."

Julie was delighted! It was the first time that JJ was positive about this idea.

When he looked up the camp and showed her what he preferred, she was surprised to see that it was a survival camp! She was excited, and a little tense because it was the first time that he had chosen to go and he had picked the most difficult camp. I felt that he would be fine, but of course I was curious to see what would happen after this big experience.

ॐॐ

Consuelo Cassotti B.S.

Sixth session (July)

JJ returned from camp very happy. He told his mom that it was the best week of his life. He was excited and spaced-out, and Julie had the impression that he needed a session to process the whole experience.

Julie was right!

Immediately, I am feeling that he needs some help to digest and transform this overwhelming experience. He is not grounded at all, very spaced-out and excited, all his pieces are scattered around him.

We work on his nervous system and joints. Because he is growing, he is taller compared to the first session.

Some Beings related to nature come to assist and help during the session. This experience made him more conscious of some memories from past lives.

A strong connection with nature emerged when he was at summer camp, and the forest helped him to re-connect with some earthy energies. I see that this experience helped a past life memory to emerge. I see him dressed as a medieval soldier, building a fire and living his life, going about a daily routine.

This camp helped him to reach more parts of himself; he is more complete, more balanced.

His mind isn't a cascade of thoughts like it was, and he doesn't need help to release thoughts like he usually does. He just needed help to organize and integrate the experience. His future self shows up again, very happy and confident. We balance the new energy and end the session. The session is over. I thank everyone.

⇄

Some weeks later, Julie sent me an email about JJ:

"Well, I have another busy day with painters and working on the house. I put JJ to work today and he is helping his uncle paint. By the way, since the last session or so his grandma and two uncles have commented about JJ, saying he is more mature. JJ's uncle said, yesterday, that he sees JJ is starting to "fill out" and get more muscles on him. It is nice to hear compliments. Years ago all I heard was: "JJ is spoiled and out of control" and I am not such a good mother! They did not understand autism at all. I don't think they ever will, but that's ok because he is better now."

Seventh session (September)

School started and JJ came for another session. The summer went well and he appeared more calm and confident.

Immediately, I can see two or three Light Beings in a line, surrounding JJ. One looks like a messenger, one seems to be one Maha Choan.

JJ's mind is more balanced and not so fast. JJ's soul is telling me that he can fly; he can be independent. A Fairy arrives, she is the same Fairy that came during another session. They start to work on his heart, it is about helping him to have a different consciousness about his way of life. He is having a shift in his consciousness in order to appreciate what he is experiencing.

Now he will pay more attention to girls, and to other "teenager stuff."

They work on his spine. The energy in this session is very feminine, very sweet. I cannot see precisely all the beings present in this session, but they are full of unconditional love, compassion and caring. They work on his DNA, and on his kidneys. They are

expanding his memory. They want to help him to see and under-
stand things with a different perspective. They open his head in the
middle and activate the pineal gland. They put something inside
to help him to be more focused, and they increase his memory up to
20%.

Today they are working on his digestive system. I am sur-
prised, because I know that Julie is very careful about his food. I
ask my Spirit Guides about this and they explain to me that he is
starting school, and sometimes JJ is probably eating food that has
poor energy. It could be processed food or non-organic that he has
at school. JJ starts to think about girls, and he is paying more at-
tention to them. I can see some faces of pretty girls that are on his
mind. Today I ask all the bodies to merge together: the physical, the
mental, the emotional and the spiritual body. The mental body was
not certain about this, but after some hesitation, it feels forgiveness
from the other parts. Now all the bodies are happy and honored to
be together, without any shame or sense of guilt from other lifetime
experiences. It is a powerful moment, and shows just how much
JJ is becoming more present and complete. Because the mental body
teamed up with the other bodies, JJ will have more memory.

A new Light Being arrives and he is a Master in mathemat-
ics. He will guide JJ when he needs help in math. He is tall and
sweet but with a serious demeanor. Also present is one who appears
to be a nanny, I'd say from the medieval times by the way that she
is dressed. The master and the nanny are currently working to sup-
port him at school. The session is over, I thank everybody.

ॐ∾

After several days, Julie shared with me that JJ had never been interested in whether or not his clothes matched,
nor paid any attention to his appearance. However, one day
earlier she saw JJ show his school pictures to his best friend,

and he said "Do you know that some girls at school said that I could be a model?"

She added that JJ was spending some time combing his hair, and she was very happy because he was acting like a kid of his age. His body was starting to show more muscle, and his demeanor was calm and confident.

Height session (given by distance November)

The session starts. I see a little imbalance on him. Some beings are working with a kind of criss-crossed energy, starting from one shoulder to the hip on the opposite side, down to the ankle and the feet, and back up from the other side.

The center where these two lines connect is the umbilicus. They work on clearing some trash and tension from his umbilicus.

They work on his breathing, not because he has an infection but because lately he isn't breathing very deeply. They suggest that I tell JJ's mother to do some breathing exercises, wherein he breathes using the whole lungs. It will be good for him. They clean the prana tube and regenerate it with prana/chi.

We recharge JJ. He is doing fine, just a little stressed. We slow down his mind, as these are old patterns that he uses when he is tired, like a safety blanket.

He is more relaxed. His mind was very tired, stressed. I advise Julie to let JJ relax sometime during the day, and play some nice music. He needs to learn how to relax himself. I work on his spine and sacrum. JJ tells me: "I am doing great!" Because of this, I believe that he really is doing fine.

They work on his hips to make them more flexible and strong. They work on his shoulders. I saw them use this combination before, and it looks like it serves to create more balance. He is having a hard time expressing himself, not because he is unable to, but because he doesn't know how to express his emotions. It is part of the teen-ager phase. They work on his throat. I see a flower that looks like a beautiful gardenia, blooming out of it.

Now it is the third eye's turn. They use some sacred symbol, and it looks like something from ancient Egypt. They awaken some knowledge and/or memories from this period. I would not be surprised if he starts to show some interest in ancient Egypt during this period of his life.

Then, I see JJ wearing military type boots. I need to ask my Spirit Guides why. They say that JJ needs to be more active. To walk in the park, in the forest, it is very important for him to find some time where he can be more with nature. They work on his torso, separating every chakra, in particular the first and the second. Now, it is the turn of the solar plexus, heart and throat. A lot of beings are working on him, from many kingdoms. JJ is very happy, he likes this moment; he feels the love and care from them. They take something off of his back to give him more space, more room to breath so that he can feel lighter.

Now all the beings make sounds and chant, in order to help integrate the vibrations. It is a nice ceremony honoring him. JJ stands up in front of everyone, very proud of himself. Everyone is here to help him recognize who he is. He looks very regal and confident. The session is over. I thank everybody.

The same day, after my session, Julie went to the school reunion, and talked to the teachers. JJ decided to create a "club" with other students.

ॐ◌ॐ

Ninth session (February)

JJ was feeling that he needed a good session. Julie asked me to help him to be more focused and energetic. He was feeling tired and stressed because of school and the many activities that he was doing.

We begin working on his stomach. It looks like he is eating some unhealthy food. We work on his liver to release toxins. I am surprised, as normally we don't need to work on his liver. They work on his joints, since he is growing again his body is stretching. Some beings work on his forehead, his third eye. They tell me that they are helping Jake to see his path with clarity. At that moment he looks kind of confused, his perception and knowledge of the future is foggy. They clear his mind, but the third eye is more confused than his mind. He looks like he is trying to understand something about his future, and he is pushing himself to see what he can do next summer, his next step at school, or the next place where he is going to live. His third eye is so full of possibilities and expectations that JJ feels confused. (This makes sense, because JJ's family is thinking about possibly moving to another State, and this means a lot of change.)

They work to make his brain sharper. They work with some energy lines in JJ's body and it looks like the shape of DNA strands. They tell me that it is for energizing him. They stretch his back again, and his whole body. Then numerous fairies surround JJ, all female. They are very sweet and in love with him. Some beings with the fairies are helping Jake to be more grounded. JJ is starting to have more feelings and hormones. Because of this, my Spirit Guides are telling me that it is time to activate some of JJ's other parts that belong to the adult field. He is growing up not only in the physical body, but all of his bodies are adjusting to the change. Some parts of him are coming during this period to merge with him, and he will feel more complete. JJ's energy is nice, well balanced and not too hyper.

My Spirit Guides say: "JJ is the son of the sun. Definitely, a move to Florida like you are planning would be very good for him, because of the sun."

JJ shows his wings, he is very proud of them. They are big and very harmonious, and he is very comfortable moving them. I can tell that he is more confident and I am so glad to see this big change. JJ's soul tells me: "Focus on my focus!"

They change the energy of his eyes so that he can see and can focus better. I feel that one of the reasons why he isn't so focused is because he has a hard time expressing himself well. I feel that because it takes so much energy, he doesn't do very well. I later notice in other children that express themselves more easily, that they require more energy than usual. Could it be that in the teenager phase it takes more energy to be certain and to explain with clarity?

Mother Theresa shows up and she works on his heart. She touches his heart and puts something inside of it. It looks like a little baby. She wants to help him to see things with new perspective.

Every being works to adjust and harmonize the changes made. It takes several minutes. I see memories from the past... He was a female wearing shoes and a dress like a Moulin Rouge dancer... then blonde hair with a ponytail. Probably two memories, one as a female, where he was very tiny and feminine, and another where he was more robust and tall, like a northern European woman.

They work with some oils on his body, and they also work on Julie's third eye.

My Spirit Guides explain that Julie is very connected to JJ. I feel that JJ is supporting Julie in this period, since she is having a hard time figuring out what to do about the move. They want to help her to have insight about her life and career.

Other memories surface, memories from past lives, parallel lives ... it looks like this time we are cleaning stuff that he doesn't need any more. Like a PC, sometimes we need to reboot and clean the files in order to give more space to others. The session is over. I thank everyone.

*Update: JJ is growing fast, and it is amazing to see how he has changed in one year. Now he is talking about a possible car purchase, since in a year and a half he will be sixteen. He is leaving the old school, and taking with him great friendships, positive experiences, some girlfriends, and a desire to become an incredible leader and compassionate young man. I am proud to be a part of his life and I cannot wait to see his successes in the future.

This is what Julie wrote me after she read this chapter:

"Because JJ was always "different" from the other kids he got teased and picked on a lot for many years. It breaks a mother's heart when their sweet child is being victimized, and the heart cries with rivers of tears for them. But it is also a lesson for them to learn from to build compassion, and you have to let that happen no matter what. That is their journey and I could not interfere too much. (Although I wanted to!) I figured if I provided a loving home for him he could conquer anything. I had to teach him to stick up for himself and say what he needed to say. It wasn't until you did the internal work at his soul level, and connected all the parts of him that he could actually do this. And then he just took off!

Consuelo Cassotti B.S.

I believe showing him his future self helped him realize how great he could be. He used to need me all the time and felt an anxiety when I wasn't around, even just last year. He has since separated from me and it is healthier for him... and me. It is wonderful to see him want this independence."

Chapter 2
"The healer that could not heal himself...until we met"

Luc was diagnosed as autistic. At the time, he was 10 years old. When he came to see me, he was not walking with much coordination. He made no eye contact, his speech was poor, a lot of "stimming" behavior* and hyperactivity.

I learned that his parents had a hard time keeping him in a public school. In fact, the teachers were starting to complain and told them that if he continued to have the same behaviors, he could no longer stay at that school.

One thing I came to realize is that, any child can understand the conversation and the words that, we use in front of them. Because of this, I prefer to use words that don't label them in a negative way. First of all, it is important for parents to begin to believe that their child is smart, and capable of understanding what is expressed by others. I understand that it can be very difficult as a parent to see this, especially when your child is very hyperactive and hard to manage... but it is still true.

As with JJ in the previous chapter, during sessions I talk with the soul of the person, and any images and conversations that I have are non-verbal.

Consuelo Cassotti B.S.

* (The term "stimming" is short for self-stimulatory behavior, sometimes also called "stereotypic" behavior. In a person with autism, stimming usually refers to specific behaviors such as flapping, rocking, spinning, or repetition of words and phrases).

First session (January)

Luc cannot stay on the massage table so he sits on a chair. Like all sessions with my clients, I focus on finding a doorway through which to connect, and I talk to the soul, reminding the person what they can do in this reality. I began the session:

Immediately, I connected with him. He is open to letting me work on him. I see/feel a lot of tension inside him. It looks like anger, but I feel that this tension doesn't belong to him. I receive information that it is his father's anger. We help Luc to release this angry energy that he has been absorbing from his father. Because it isn't his own emotion, he has a hard time recognizing and handling it.

I ask Luc's soul how long he wants to be this way, and he answers me "Soul to soul"…"A couple of years." We work on the nervous system, as it is a weakness in him. I work to tune the Nervous System from the spine. It looks like a guitar string that needs to be tuned. It takes several minutes.

His mind his always busy, it is spinning incredibly. My Spirit Guides suggest that it would help to let Luc use more colors and paint, to keep the mind busy but at a nice pace.

Luc shows his wings. Only one wing begins to show, on the left. It is a very small wing for his age. His right shoulder looks physically unbalanced, and this shoulder has no wing. Luc is taking his right shoulder up in an unnatural way.

Meanwhile, I continue working on him and I notice that Luc is sending my healing session to someone else, not present in the room.

(Regular conversation) I ask Luc's mother: "Does Luc have siblings?" because I see a tall young male, and he is connected to Luc and Luc is sending him some healing energy. I describe the picture that I see and Luc's mother says: "He is his big brother, Ryan!" In some way, Luc was helping his big brother.

I decide to help Luc to be clearer and less connected to anyone but himself. He needs some help to clear this. I call the Archangel Michael to clear all the emotional cords attached to Luc. We clear all emotions from him. He is looking more balanced and calm. We ground him so that he can be more present and in his body. The session is over. I thank everyone.

One thing that I have noticed in sensitive children is that they are like a sponge. They can absorb any emotions from the people that surround them. The difficulty for them is to manage and clear themselves of these emotions. They don't understand these emotions, since they don't belong to them, but they still experience them. Energy work is very helpful to clear and release stress and emotions.

When I speak of clearing "energetic emotional cords", what I mean is that I clear emotionally, the connection between people. Many times, people are connected not only because of love, but because of a sense of guilt, shame, an-

Consuelo Cassotti B.S.

ger, dependency, etc. We are more connected than we realize. The connection cannot be broken, but it can be made more neutral. This permits people to have better relationships, and to stand on their own.

ॐ❧

Feedback from Luc's mother: "When we were driving home, he looked tired and he fell asleep. The next day he was a little hyper, but in the days that followed, I noticed that he was less anxious, less overactive. At school he is calmer, and the teachers say that it looks like it is going to be easier to handle him".

ॐ❧

Second session (February)

Today I see Light Beings working on Luc giving a "maintenance session", fast and easy. Observing them, I see they are raising his vibration. They are energetically changing some parts of his body because of the new vibration. A pure maintenance session is fast, more focused on raising the vibration and changing the parts to fit the new vibration. He is very open to energy work.

This time he has not emotionally attached to any member of his family; he doesn't heal anyone else by distance. I am happy to see that Luc is receiving the healing session just for himself! This is a big step.

We create a filter in his ears so that he can better handle sound. Now, grounding and slowing down his thoughts... The session is over. I thank everyone.

Sometimes I prefer not to explain some information in front of the child. Because of this, after the session, I send an email to Luc's Mother: *"I have noticed that Luc's interaction is very good. The first time he was sending help to his brother, transforming his father's anger, and he was probably helping you too. This time he was more focused on himself, he was not spreading it around (energetically speaking.) He worked only for himself and he was receiving what he really needs. During the second session, I was feeling his desire to be more independent. His wings are not yet ready, but he is working on it."*

She answered back, that she was seeing some small changes in his behavior, like being more flexible to change, calmer, and more coordinated.

Third session (given by distance, March)

The first thing I notice is that Luc is surrounded by a yellow energy; his aura is completely yellow. This color is related to the mind and to the solar plexus. I see that he is releasing some energy from his solar plexus. I can hear some angels playing (the) harp, they are explaining to me that they are very connected to Luc and that they are here today to help him with this music, so that he may relax and rest more.

In fact, in this period he looks tired, like he needs more time to rest during the day. Luc tells me that he is excited about something. I don't know if it is a project at school, a birthday, or something else, but he is preparing himself for this particular positive event.

They work on his back. They tell me that his back is the key to a lot of issues. We work on his back, in his shoulder area. It looks like the flow of energy in his back is stuck. If he does some stretching of his back it could be helpful. In fact, he is happy that we are taking care of his back. I work on his spine, and on all the nerves connected to his spine. During this work one of my hands is attracted to his throat, and I help him with this. It feels as though something is caught in his throat, and I cough for him (I am helping with his communication.) I believe that after today his language skills are going to improve. I send him the color blue, a very calming blue. I sent him other calming colors of blue and purple too, they are very powerful.

I work on his "prana tube", clearing it and sending pranic energy. The prana tube looks like a crystal tube, in the mid-line of the body. I have noticed that the clearer it is, the more energized the client is, and the better the organs work.

He has something going on in his mind concerning his father. Luc is worried about him. He explains to me that he worries about the way his father is. I tell him that he doesn't need to take care of his father. His father is a big guy.

Luc requests to have his third eye be more open; this will help him to perceive the future and better understand the next steps. Because he asks for this we do it. Next we work on the link between his heart and his throat. Luc wants to speak with his heart; he wants to speak what he feels. He is an incredibly sweet soul, and very powerful.

I ask him: "what else do you need?"–He answers: "to release some stress".

Luc is like a sponge. Until he learns how to shield himself better, he will always absorb stuff from others. He will need to be helped, through energy sessions, to clear himself of what he has absorbed. Luc expressed "I like to take care of other people." I explain to him that it is ok to love others, especially his family, but he needs to take care of himself first. If he were more balanced, his family would be happier. It is hard for him to think about himself, he isn't selfish. I want to help him accept the idea that it is important at this time to take care of himself first. We work on his heart, now the energy starts to expand everywhere around him and inside him. It is a very relaxing moment, and he enjoys it too.

It is difficult for him to accept the idea that if he is happy, his family is happy. In his mind he believes that he needs to take care of everyone else. I suggest that his mother tell him sometimes that it is ok to take care of himself (it occurs to me that he is coping like his mother, she always puts others first.) It is incredible the way the energy is expanding, he has a strong energy. I check his back and the flow in his back is wonderful. Everything looks fine. The session is over. I thank everyone.

When I emailed the recorded session, I suggested to his mother the use of colors like blue or green for his blanket or sheets, perhaps a blue t-shirt. I am feeling that, this would help him, to feel more calm and relaxed through color therapy.

శ్రీ శ్రీ

Fourth session (given by distance–April)
Luc needed to calm his mind and to be more present and focused. His mother asked me to help him desire to eat more varieties of food. Luc is very sensitive to food.

He seems better every time. I feel that he is tired, but also excited at the same time. "We recharge his battery" and clean him of other people's stuff. He has a hard time taking care of himself first. Luc is very sensitive to other people and the environment.

Consuelo Cassotti B.S.

We work on stretching his back, we clean his throat and his nervous system. I notice an energy bridge between his heart and his throat. I have the feeling that he is looking to communicate with his heart more than before.

I plant the seed in his mind that he can be who he wants. I change that part of his belief system that says that he cannot change, to believe that he can be anything he wants. The session is over. I thank everyone.

After the first week, Luc's mother informed me that sometimes he needed few days to adjust to the new energy session, but Luc was doing well.

෴

Fifth session (May)
I asked Luc what he wanted from this session, he requested to be able to ride his bike with more coordination.

The session starts. We work on the digestive system and the joints. He allows me to communicate with him at the soul level. I work on his self-esteem. It seems that he starts to believe what I am saying to him. It is a very good sign.

The way that he looks at me shows me that something is starting to click. I have the impression that he is changing his belief system about himself. We help him to have more confidence. I talk to him about something that is challenging, but that he likes to do. He likes to ride his bike. I tell him that the more he is present in his body and believes in himself, the better he will be able to ride his bike. Today is about building his self-esteem, his confidence.

Because I don't see his wings, I think that he needs a little more time to trust and feel more confident. The session is over. I thank everyone.

Feed back from Luc's mother:

There are so many positive changes happening with Luc and she claims they all started with these sessions. She said "it definitely, without a doubt ... started when you started working with him."

These may seem like trivial situations but when you have a child with special needs, it is a very big deal.

☞ ☜

Some weeks after the session, Luc's mother sent me an email about specific good results:

"Last November, Luc's grade school had performed a musical for the parents. Luc was not able to stand up with the other kids and participate, so the aides put him in a chair next to the other kids who were standing on the bleachers. He had to have his shoes off (a sensory thing) and sit on the chair with his legs crossed. He was able to sit there and look around, but did not sing or interact. Now, this May, they are doing another similar play for the parents. Luc did not want to sit in the chair this time. He wanted to stand up and sing with the other kids (with his shoes on). I was watching and filming this event for my husband. We are very excited to see him want to be like the other kids and not have special accommodations. He is also going to sing!!!

The teachers have all reported back with positive changes within the last few months and also claim that he probably will not need an aide with him next school year. He follows the class schedules. He needs less and less support as he is doing more independently. I might add that he had a very tough time at school the first half of the year. By December I debated whether or not I should even keep him in school. The teachers even commented that they were not sure if they could keep him there at school with his behavior problems.

That has all changed now.

I had purchased a special bike for Luc late last year. Luc has always struggled with muscle control and brain function in the past, so bike riding and swinging on a swing were extremely difficult for him to accomplish. A month ago, out of the blue Luc got on his bike and started to ride it. Now Luc asks to go outside and ride his bike on nice days. I now have to run to stay up with him, and he even slows down to wait for me to catch up. Luc rarely asked to go outside and play until now. Now, I am happily trying to figure out how to keep up with him!!!

Luc has always struggled with change in his environment. This is very common with autism. Last year we pulled up carpet in the family room and put in hardwood floors. Luc was upset for months over this and would get so angry he would throw things at the wood floor to damage it. That has now stopped. This Spring we even removed a play set, as well as a hot tub in the backyard, with little to no outbursts. His outbursts are more under control and that makes life easier on all of us.

Luc is also eating a wider variety of foods. A few years ago, he could only tolerate beef, chicken, and water. His diet was very limited for many years. Even a teaspoon of broth was too much for him to handle ... . It would blow him away. Now he is eating lunchmeat and brown rice for lunch, and I continue to experiment with new foods he seems to be able to tolerate now. This is huge because it can be very difficult to go somewhere without packing special foods. Also, living with the fear that if he eats something that doesn't agree with him, his behaviors might be off for days. That's no fun!"

Sixth session (June)

I started the session after some requests from Luc's mother. More foods, more new articulated words, and Luc said that he wants to use his bike more. His mother and I asked him if he preferred to lie down on the massage table, and he agreed.

I begin the session. Finally his wings are complete! They are very small, but well made. He is more in control, with more clarity about his life. He allows me to give him a good session. He is very open to cooperation. I work on his digestive system and nervous system. He is more balanced and focused than the month before, but I want to reinforce this. Now his energy is more balanced and he is more focused. He asks to be able to ride is bicycle with better co-ordination. He is growing and starting to produce more hormones. As I was clearing his emotional connection with his mother, he says loudly:

(Regular conversation) Luc turns his face to his mother, makes eyes contact with her and he says: "Mom I love you!"

Today, he is very cooperative. He handles a twenty minute long session for the first time!

Consuelo Cassotti B.S.

The session is over. I thank everyone...

࿇

Seventh session (July)

Maintenance session. Like I explained before, I call it a maintenance session, as during the session I don't receive particular information, but we take care of the "regular stuff." Just like with a car; change the oil, rotate the tires, add some gasoline. Normally, it doesn't seem that we go very deep. I have the impression that it is a session wherein we support the changes from the session before, as it sometimes takes time and assistance to integrate them.

࿇

Eighth session (August)

Luc's mother Mary, Julie, and I talked about how much these children are affected by mercury, heavy metals, and yeast. Luc is using only very natural medications/supplements and he is eating well enough, but his system can only release some of this "stuff." Because of this I decided to see if my Spirit Guides and I could do more to clean his body.

I begin the session and immediately understand that the priority is to work on his brain and help both sides to integrate better. We work on the nervous system, his spine, and we start to do regular maintenance. I ask if we can work on yeast and mercury, and the reply is: "Yes." They are telling me how much is in his body, and they suggest how much we take care of today. They tell me: "The liver isn't too toxic, but we can clean it too". Spirit Guides explain that the crux of his problem is with the food in his stomach. Because of this we alkalinized the gastric acid. With this done everything expands more!

(Regular conversation) Luc's mother asks "Can you tell me how much of the toxins in his body are from his baby shots?"

They answer: "Not too much is left." I feel that Luc's body seems to have released most of these toxins. One big priority is his digestive system. We work with Luc to increase his variety of foods. We work on his stamina. I explain to him how it is good to be more grounded, particularly when he is riding his bike. He likes the idea and this construct works.

He shows me his future self... confident, tall and well built. He looks like a twenty year—old boy. He said that the reason he has chosen to be this way is because it was necessary for his family. This helped them to be what they are now, to think in the way that they now think.

We clear the emotional cords. At the end of the session they want to integrate his knowledge. The session is over. I thank everyone.

Feed back from Julie, who has the occasion to talk with Luc's mother the day after the session.

Julie said that Mary was so very happy!

The night after the session, Luc came home from the session and insisted on fixing the toilet with the plunger. He locked himself in the bathroom and then came out smiling, saying he fixed it! He did.

His father was present, and he is starting to see more results in his son too."

అ౼ళ

Consuelo Cassotti B.S.

Some days after the session, I needed to help Luc by distance; he had more "stimming" behavior and was a little grumpier than usual.

Normally it takes one to two weeks for Luc to adjust completely to the energy work. A lot of autistic children have a problem with mercury and heavy metals due to vaccinations. The body has a hard time managing the amount. I have worked on other children like Luc, to free the body of yeast, mercury and heavy metals, and I realized that their bodies can handle the cleansing pretty well, but the parents have a hard time managing their children. They become less present and moody. The body needs time and energy to adjust to the change. This is the reason why I don't take too much yeast, mercury, or heavy metals out of the body at one time now, and I advise the parents about the "side-effects." Indeed, Luc showed some difficulty being present after this work.

Luc was also playing with video games every night and I believe that affected him a great deal. It was as though he was never disconnected from the video game, even when he wasn't playing.

Some of Luc's old behavior patterns from years ago showed up again. I believe that part of this behavior is because we removed a lot of toxins from him last session. The baby vaccinations, plus the yeast and mercury were a lot for him to handle in one session

I asked his mother to find something else that Luc can do before bedtime. His mind needs to slow down before going to sleep.

Most of the children are very affected by computer and video games, their minds start to spin and they never rest completely.

෨ඁ෬

Eighth session (end of August)
Luc's mother and I, have decided that Luc needed a session in three weeks, because the school was starting. He had a difficult month, and I wanted to be sure that he would have some help at the beginning of school.

We work immediately on balancing the spinal cord. We balance all the chakras to the mid-line and we start to work on his third eye (front of head.) We help both sides of his brain to work more as a team. We regenerate the stomach wall, the colon and the liver.

We ground him and then ground him again. We want to help him to be positive and happy for the first days at school next week. He still has a hard time believing that he can be in charge of himself. He tells me (soul to soul) that he wants to go to school and show how much he has grown this summer, but he is hesitant because he is not so confident in what he can do. We work on his joints; he is growing in his back and nervous system.

We do energy work in four different points at the base of his head and neck. We work also on his spine, his sacrum and his diaphragm. He shows us his wings. They are small, but well built and a little transparent and ethereal.

We find a blockage in his throat that is related to his anxiety and frustration. We came back to the grounding, and I explain to him that the more present he is in his body, the more easily he can ride his bike and enjoy other physical activities.

Consuelo Cassotti B.S.

His skin is releasing some toxins from the last session. His brain (that now works in regular waves and not so fast like the first sessions), is releasing some "trash"... like ideas, pictures, images. I believe that was part of his memory of the video games. We work on his ears; he still has a problem with some sounds. We end the session with some energy work. Luc allows us to work on him for twenty minutes. The session is over. I thank everyone.

Feedback from Luc's mother:
"Luc has had a great week at school, just like it never ended. Thanks!"
Follow up:
Luc has had a great two weeks of school.

ॐ✑

Ninth Session (September)
With great pleasure, I was listening to Luc's mother explain her concerns about Math. She explained that Luc was struggling in math. At the moment he was in a "special class" only for math, and she believed that the program level in this class was too low for him. She told me that if he showed that he was doing better, the teachers could move him into a regular math class. She also told me that she would love to see him make some friends.

Immediately we work on his lungs and other parts of his body. I ask about Luc's difficulty socializing. My Spirit Guides inform me that he can only socialize with people that have a role, or a specific job in his life. Those that he feels more of a relationship with, like teachers, aides, me... Luc is still in the period where he needs to shield himself from being too close (emotionally) to others.

40

Other children are too full of emotions and energy, and this over-whelms him. He isn't ready to be so involved with other children, but adults with this kind of role he can handle. When he starts to have some filters he will be ready to have new relationships.

His heart is very calm and beautiful. I don't see any anxiety. Emotionally he is very well, very balanced. We work on his spine and nervous system. His digestive system is better, from what I can see he can eat a greater variety of food. His joints need some work because he is still growing. He tells me that he prefers boys to girls for friends (I think that it is normal for his age.)

They also work on Luc's mother. They work on her back and her wings. I ask Luc if he can explain why he is having a hard time in Math. Luc shows me that the reason why he feels stuck in math is because he didn't completely understand something, there is some small hole in his learning of a math concept and because of this he cannot progress further in math.

The session is over. I thank everyone.

ॐ ॐ

Tenth Session (given by distance–November)

Mary decided to take the "One Blessing" some months before. She decided to give the blessing to Luc every day. She asked me to check to see if it is ok to continue every day, or if it is better to slow down.

We start immediately to work on his nervous system; Luc is having a hard time. We begin by helping him to relax. We then help him to ground himself better. They work on slowing down his brain waves. I ask him: "How are you?" He answers "GOOD!"

We work on his stomach. He is releasing toxins, breathing deeply, and relaxing more. They are energizing him; they are focused on his legs. I ask my Spirit Guides "Why?" They say because he needs help to make better use of his legs. Luc shows me *that he has some tension because of school. This is part of his adjustment to the school program, he is doing fine.*

I ask my Spirit Guide if the blessing that his mom is giving him everyday is right for him. The answer is yes. We are finished working on his body. We harmonize the energy work before closing the session. It takes several minutes. The session is over. I thank everybody...

&⁓&

Eleventh Session (December) I

I start the session. Immediately, I hear some information for Luc's mother. They say that she needs to rest more. Lately she doesn't take care of herself. It also looks like when she is resting her mind remains active.

(Regular conversation) I explain to her what I just heard and she agrees.

They decide to clear her mind, and in the meantime they work on Luc. They work on his digestive system like it was a priority. He has some acidity, and it is necessary to alkalinize his stomach. Two or three days ago he ate something that created this situation. They suggest trying some hot water with lemon on an empty stomach in the morning for several days. Luc asks me to check his heart. His heart is full of energy. I don't understand why he asked me to check it. Luc says: "I want to love more; I want more energy in my heart"

We work on the Nervous System and various organs and systems. Luc says: "I want to be an inventor when I grow up."

What occurs to me is that Luc has the ability to see from a different perspective, and this will help him.

Luc says: "My mom will be proud of me!" I can see different beings that are working with him today, and they are very tall and slim. They are carrying knowledge from ancient times. They start to work on me too. I wasn't expecting this! There are two specific beings resembling a couple from Babylon. The male is the master of the knowledge. He will help Luc to be more present and to better express what he has in his mind. Luc is well supported by kind and loving beings. They work on the top of his head. They want to help him expand his knowledge, his logical mind. They balance his chakras. Today it looks like they are preparing him to better understand and express his knowledge. It's as though everything was locked up inside, and now it is time to let this knowledge come out. Luc is reacting very well to this session. I ask him about the possibility of having more relationships. He answers: "Next spring." There is a boy that he likes. Not with dark hair, but kind of blonde and he is a short boy.

(Regular conversation) I describe to Luc's mother what I see; she says that she knows this boy.

This boy has the right energy for Luc. The session is over. I thank everyone

⇘⇛

Consuelo Cassotti B.S.

Twelfth Session (January)

Luc's mother noticed some imbalances, she is very sensitive too and this helps her to pick up on the changes. Luc is very sensitive to the full moon and I feel that a big shift is coming for him this year. I believe that every time there is an energy shift in the planet or some natural event, these children are affected by it. They are so sensitive and connected to everything in the energy grid, more than we realize.

Luc is very unbalanced, not very grounded. His nervous system needs help. Normally I see him more aligned, today he isn't. He let us see his heart, I feel that what Luc has tried to do is open his heart, but he cannot figure out when to let it be open and when to close it. He needs to understand how to shield himself. It is difficult for him to figure out how to handle being in harmony. His mother tells me that another healer worked on his heart with BodyTalk technique last week.

Probably he is still adjusting to this work. His energy today is very chaotic and not harmonic. Everywhere I look, I see the same situation. I believe that the energy at the beginning of 2012 is also part of these movements in Luc. We work in many places. Luc is taking in a lot of information. He is like an antenna that is receiving information, never stopping. In this period everyone is receiving more information, but these children are more exposed to this energy.

(A lot of sensitive people are having a hard time filtering and shielding themselves from this energy, and receiving the knowledge without feeling overwhelmed).

Some fairies arrive to work on both shoulders and his arms. I asked if we could help his digestive system. They say: "He will always be sensitive to food, but we can work on this." I also ask if

Luc's mother Mary needs some work, like in the last session. They tell me: "She is doing better now. It isn't necessary today." The session is over. I thank everyone.

Feedback:
The day after the session, the school organizes a folk dance with the children. Mary was recording the dance at the gym with her phone. She sent me the video clip and I had a hard time finding Luc. He was doing everything the others kids did. He stood on the line with the boys, facing the girls. He gave his hand to the girl in front of him, and he followed the rhythm of the drum with his feet. The only difficulty he had was in hearing the loud sounds of the other classes. He was covering his ears because the sound hurt them. I was amazed!

తా∽

Short session given by distance (January)
At the end of January, 20 days later, I did a distance session, because his mother noticed that he was having a hard time relaxing.

His nervous system is very tense. It looks like one teacher is affecting his balance. She is loaded with emotions, and Luc is picking them up from her. It could be a new teacher, or an old teacher with a different energy. They tell me to slow down with the blessing, that he shouldn't have it every day now. He tells me that he loves this blessing from his mother, but it is a little too much at this moment. It could be that Mary has helped him to reach a point where he has enough of this incredible energy, and he needs to back off a bit with the blessings.

Luc starts to talk to me. He tells me that all the kids that are having sessions with me are connected to one another, and I am the bridge. I ask him if it is ok to come this Friday to have a session in person and he answers affirmatively. I can see that Luc is more relaxed. He smiles at me and I feel that he is doing better now. He points to his stomach, and I receive the information that is related to the emotions at his school. I feel the sadness that belongs to someone else. He feels sorry for her. The session is over. I thank everyone.

Feedback:

Luc's mother is unable to discover whether or not any teachers are going through a difficult experience. She is a very private person and the teachers don't know about this energy session. Luc was doing better.

ॐ∽

Thirteenth Session (February)

Our sessions were becoming longer, around 20 or 30 minutes. Luc can sit or lie down on the table. In this particular time he seemed a little confused and not completely focused. His mother cannot explain what was going on.

I start the session. I see a big pillar of light going through different parts of his body. Luc is full of energy, and he is expanding. I feel that it is the result of his mother's blessings. He shows me his heart. It is very confused, very chaotic. We help him to find more clarity. We replace his heart energetically, and he seems to easily allow this. I see a female figure with long blonde hair, and she is very sad. Luc is absorbing this sadness and he is trying to heal her. Luc's wings are very big and beautiful. This is a metaphor for Luc becoming more independent and free to be who he wants to be. My Spirit Guides are confirming that Luc is a healer. I don't see him working as a healer in the future, as he wants to do something more creative, but he is a natural healer.

We work on his spine, to release the tension. He is producing more hormones. He starts having feelings that he cannot explain because they are a result of his hormones. We clear him, and we clear the emotional cords. I have never seen Luc be so full of emotions and emotional garbage. We work on his joints and his muscles and organs. I hold space and let him release even more. I ask to create a "bubble" around him that will help him to shield himself from other people's emotions. We finish the session. I thank everyone.

Luc's grandfather died a week after the session. Mary said that Luc was very different from his usual self, and when they went to see her father when he was close to passing, Luc told her that he could see his grandpa's angels close to him. Family members looked at him when he said this, and he said immediately "I am kidding!"

Mary had the impression that Luc was helping his grandpa to leave, and her to mourn his death. Lately, Luc has been less focused, not very grounded, and tired. He was taking care of his family. Because of this, Mary decided to have a session for herself. She knows how much she can affect her son, and how he will try to take care of her. When her mother was dying, Mary promised her that she would take care of her father. Luc probably felt her sense of responsibility, and he helped her with it until the end.

Consuelo Cassotti B.S.

Mary's session (March)

Mary's session went very well. She really needed to release emotions and recharge her batteries. She was very open and relaxed during the session and she was able to let go of a lot of stress. She released also some sadness related to her father.

༂∾ঔ

Fourteen Session (March)

Luc seamed to (be) doing better at school.

Immediately I feel Luc is lighter. It looks like this phase is complete. Luc said to me: "Finally, done!" I see some yellow light coming from his shoulders, like an expansion. I believe that he is finished taking care of his family. He is happy that his mother is taking care of herself. His Angels/Spirit Guides smile at him and say that they are very proud of him. He did a good job! (I think that they are talking about the family issues.)

They work on his spine, nervous system, and eyes. They want to help him to see things in a different way, and his eyes become golden in color. His heart is perfect. Better than last time... no comparison. We work on his solar plexus. I explain to him that when he feels the need for stimming he needs to breathe deeply.

Luc tells me that he is afraid to grow up, afraid to change. He said that nobody can understand him like his mom does. I can feel that this is the reason why he is afraid to grow up, because of his uncertainty about his relationship with his mother. He isn't sure that their relationship will stay the way that it is. He needs to find a good reason to grow up.

(Regular conversation) Luc says to his mother: "Mom, I love you!"

I explain to him that when he grows up he can have friends, drive a car, and he can continue to protect his mother if he wants. Then I see beautiful colors... rainbow colors, good expansion and good energy.

Luc tells me that he wants to be a pilot when he grows up.

(Regular conversation) I ask Mary: Does he show some interest in airplanes or any vehicles that fly?—she cannot say.

I don't understand what kind of pilot he is talking about, but it is nice to have him send me a message about the future. We finish working. The session is over. I thank everyone.

ॐॐ

Fifteen Session (April)

Luc is more interactive. He tells me what he wants from his session and he chooses his preference for chair or table. He is doing very well, more balanced and relaxed.

I start the session. His mind is spinning very fast, like an infinity symbol. They work on his brain, his spine, and his sacrum. We work on his body, and I clear some stuff from different parts of his body. I feel that it is easier to be in his body this year. Sean's soul tells me "I can be more in my body!"

(Regular conversation) Luc says: "My head hurts." We work on his head. Luc smiles. He is cleansing fast and easy.

For several minutes his body releases all the things that Luc has accumulated from the environment, from other people, from food. His body is more capable of managing toxins and emotions. I can see "stuff" coming out throughout the session. I smell fried food. Mary admits that he has had some fast food today.

They update him with new information and help him to become more aware of the knowledge that he has already. It takes several minutes. I feel that the memory of who he can become is a little foggy, like he has forgotten about it, so I remind him. I also remind him to ground himself better in his body. He is listening, he just forgot to do it. The session is over. I thank everyone.

࿇

Sixteen session (May)

Luc's mother asked me if I could help him more in math, and with some friends.

She told me that they plan to go on vacation soon and he will be at the pool a lot. The water has a magical effect on these children. I think it is because it helps the nervous system to relax.

The session starts, they work on his head. I ask to have a master or Spirit Guide that can help him to do better in math. My Spirit Guides agree. His stomach has better energy, and he is expanding. I feel that he can eat a greater variety of foods. I know that just a spoonful of something can affect him. They work on his liver and I am surprised to hear an Angel says: "No more French fries!"

(Regular conversation) When I express to Luc's Mother the request, she admits that, lately, he was eating French fries every day. Luc, with his voice says: "I love French fries!"

We work on his joints because he is growing a lot lately. We stretch his back. I check to see if Luc has a problem with the chlorine in the pool. He is doing fine. He shows me that sometimes he has a hard time managing a relationship with other children. He doesn't know what to do. He prefers to avoid any situation where he needs to have contact with other children. He can also absorb other emotions. He feels tense when he has to start a new relationship. He shows me a picture of two children, a male and a female. These kids are fine with him, and he doesn't have any problem interacting with them. He is growing, not just physically, but experientially. Before, he would have experiences, but he would forget about them. Now when he experiences something, he archives it and holds on to the experience. Through these experiences he is beginning to grow.

I remind him about himself and he answers me: "I am doing my best." This is good because it feels like he is aware of his path. I feel him becoming more relaxed about his mother, it seems he doesn't need to take care of her so much now. I am glad because now he can focus more on himself.

I ask a Spirit Guide to help Luc to read better, and with better comprehension.

His hearing, such as his reaction to the loud sound, is still something that bothers him and we work on this. The session is over. I thank everyone.

After the session, I suggested to Mary that she could invite the two children that Luc showed me to come over, perhaps with their parents to create a moment outside of school, where they could see each other. It could be nice to choose a place like a park, where they might interact freely.

さ～ら

Consuelo Cassotti B.S.

In June, at the end of the school year, Mary showed me a class picture taken that day. She said that in last year's picture he was on the side, not singing. In the current photo, Luc was sitting in the center of the picture, singing! Of course, during the singing he would sometimes cover his ears because the noise was too much, but he was singing just like everyone else. His talking is becoming more articulate, and today he passed two tests at school.

❧ ❧

Seventeen session (July)

Luc has decided to be in the massage table instead of the usual chair. His mother sat on his side and they were smiling at each other. Luc was calm.

I start the session. Immediately, I can see that Luc looks and feels very happy. I ask him why, and he explains that he is happy because school would be over tomorrow. He says that he would be less stressed now. He likes to have some free time.

For some reason, he is telling me that he wants to be a fireman. I like the fact that he is starting to project himself into the future, and it is a good sign. I have a positive impression about this summer. He is starting to be more open to changes and to having new experiences.

We work a little on his mind. We want to decrease his sensitivity to sound. They work on his mind and his energy is good. We don't need to clean him too much. We finish working. The session is over. I thank everyone.

*Update: Today Luc continues to make improvements. I am very happy that he and his parents trust me, and have decided to continue working with me. I truly believe that all these results are possible because he has always used natural remedies and medications that make it possible for my energy work to be effective. Before I met him, Luc had a Naturopathic Doctor and a BodyTalk practitioner working on him for some years. I helped to take him "out of the box" and build his self-esteem, and show him the possibility that he can be who he wants. No more labels or notions that he can never be better, or that he can't become a man with his own way of using his incredible skills. Luc will always be special, because he learned how to see things differently. He will always be a sensitive person, and in his case a natural healer.

I also believe that when Luc integrates more fruits and vegetables into his diet, he will have another big shift. Working on his digestion and on his family's food habits, will lead him to become (or to merge with) the future self that I met during our sessions. I am so happy that he allows me to be part of his path in this life.

Chapter 3
"The girl with an immense heart, who didn't know that she could be more grown up"

Violet's parents brought her to me when she told them that she didn't feel happy anymore. They are very caring and open-minded people, willing to listen and try something non-invasive to help their daughter, without the addition of more medication. Violet was twenty years old, and she was always carrying a Japanese Anime Manga Series stuffed hero-doll, Naruto. Doctors said that Violet was bipolar, schizophrenic and autistic, with some anxiety. When we met, she was very sweet and polite, but spoke and acted like a sweet twelve <u>years</u> (twelve-year-old) old girl.

Her parents wanted to try my sessions, rather than give her more medication. In fact, their goal was to gradually diminish her medications. Her diet was good and she liked healthy food. She was integrating salads, veggies, and fruits very well with other food.

First session (August)
Violet was very open to work with me.

Consuelo Cassotti B.S.

I start the session. Violet has good energy and she is very vital. They help her to clear her mind of old memories and information that she doesn't need anymore. She has an incredible memory, but like a PC that is too busy with many files, it needs to be cleaned. She is very open and we start a soul-to-soul conversation. She tells me that she is afraid of not loving others enough. She lives with a lot of anxiety and emotion over this. I tell her that first she needs to love her-self then she can feel complete. After this she can give her love to other people. It is very important for her to recognize that she is important too. I explain to her the metaphor of the glass of water; when it is full she can give water to other people, but first she needs to have a full glass of water. Immediately she answers: "Good, this means that I can make two glasses!"

I feel that she means she can love even more people. I asked her: "How long do you want to be this way?" Violet looked at me with surprise and said: "I didn't know that I could be different!" She is full of fear and my body is shaking because of it. We work on her mind to help her to clear her emotions. She shows me pictures of her at the age of eight years. She tells me: "This is the period when I didn't want to be a female anymore."

(Regular conversation) I gave this information to her mother. She explained that the pressure at school was very high for Violet during that particular period.

I perceived that in Violet's class there was one particular boy who was a very good student, and made very good grades. She started to compare herself to him and began to think that the reason why she wasn't such a good student was because she was female.

(Regular conversation) I explain to her mother what I saw. She is telling me that she remembers this period in the second grade, when Violet was obsessed with a particular boy. Violet then adds with her voice "Evan!" I am feeling that Violet now recognizes that this isn't true, and she can be a female...

I don't know where this will take us, but certainly a blocked emotion has been released. I told her that she is a beautiful girl and that her dad loves her, and she smiles.

Today we also clear her of mercury and other metals, just a little because it can be overwhelming for her if we do too much at once. I explain to her that her doll has superpowers, but she does too. She has powers within she just needs to begin to reach them. Her doll is always connected to her, even when she doesn't carry it with her. The doll will always be where she needs it and available to help. Yes! She listens to me, she is very focused but still cautious about me.

I ask her: "May I see your wings?" She looks at me timidly, and I feel that she isn't ready to open herself completely to me. It is her first session. I tell her to breathe deeply, this way she will be able to hear better, and express herself more easily.

They work on a particular point on her head. I cannot understand. I ask if I can have some clarification. They tell me that it is not about what she hears from the outside, but mostly what she hears inside of her head. They say that she needs more of a filter. She hears many voices and she is having a hard time finding her own voice. I have the impression that she could be more telepathic, and she is having a hard time distinguishing her own thoughts from those of others.

We want to help her to have more filters so that she can feel better. They tell me that we can do a little today but we will need other sessions. We also work on another part of her head; the energetic points connected to her speech patterns (the back of the head, close to the neck and mandible.) It looks as though they are a little disconnected.

(Regular conversation) Violet complains about her head, she feels some pressure. We finish working on her head. She feels better. The session is finished. I thank everyone.

Feedback:

Violet's mother called to give me an update. She said that immediately after her session Violet was less anxious. She also noted that before the session on a scale from 1 to 10, Violet's anxiety was a 10. Immediately following the session, and in the days after, her anxiety dropped to a 4. Several days later, her mother sent me an email stating that Violet was painting more than usual and she was looking happier.

꙳

Second Session (September)

Violet's mother confirmed that Violet was doing well, she was calmer and happier every day.

I start the session. Today is really about being present and being more grounded, it looks like she asked for this. I see some beings work on her feet repeatedly.

I feel that she sees and behaves as though everything is black and white, and she has a hard time understanding anything in be-

tween. Bad words or good words, if she hears someone say something that isn't very nice, she has a hard time letting go of it. For Violet words are important. When somebody says something, Violet thinks that it is true. She doesn't understand that some people speak without paying too much attention to what they say, or whether it is superficial or false. It is difficult for her to understand that some people just open their mouths and speak just to be talking.

Metaphorically, I see Violet put her foot on the other side of the line where there are unkind words, and she looks at me. I encourage her to do it and I explain to her that it is ok. Sometimes people use unkind words, in a different gradation between black and white, bad and good. Now it looks like she is starting to explore this possibility. It is a learning process for her.

I explain to her that she shouldn't pay attention to the unkind words that people sometimes use. These words are not so important. Some people use bad words only because it is easy. I can see that for years she has recorded these words in her mind and when she is stressed these memories come up, and she feels ashamed of herself, because she has these expressions she has heard locked away in her mind.

Today my job is to help her understand that there is nothing so bad about this (the more she forces herself not to use them, the more these words create stress in her—if she learns to let go of these thoughts then she won't store them in her memory banks.)

Violet sent me a picture of her frightened and alone, and I cannot understand what it is about.

(Regular conversation) I explain and ask her mother, Violet's mother couldn't recall a moment like this. I ask to clear this trauma and release any worries. She breathes like she is releasing some heaviness. Violet then said: " I am feeling weird".

Consuelo Cassotti B.S.

I ask if we could increase her focus so that she could read better and vocalize more. They tell me that it is something that needs to be increased slowly, and so we will repeat this at different times during the session. We work on her eyes. She doesn't need to wear reading glasses, but lately they tell me, her eyes are tired and have less energy. It is one of the reasons why she has stopped reading as much. We clear all memories of fear from her skin, her pores, her cells...

(Regular conversation) Because she starts to hug her doll more tightly, I ask her: "Are you ok?" Violet answers: "I am just terrified!" I am feeling that it is a big step for her, and her doll is like her "security blanket."

I send her love and I explain to her soul that it isn't important whether she has the doll with her or not, she will be equally protected. I also reassure her: "You can hold the doll, nobody wants to pressure you to give up your doll."

Because I see an image of her with other teen-agers I tell her "You have a lot of friends."

Violet answers me: "Yes, but Naruto is different. It is only with him (the doll) that I feel I can talk about everything. With Naruto I can share any emotion."

I answer her: "If you need Naruto, it is ok."

Immediately she feels the urge to clarify: "Naruto doll isn't my baby, but my friend!"

I have the feeling that she sees her Naruto doll on the same level as herself. I explain to her: "You are powerful like Naruto, you both have superpowers."

(Regular conversation) Violet said: "I don't know how to describe it. I just need to hug him!" I smile at her when I answer: "It is ok to hug him."

We work on harmonizing the new vibration. She did a great job. The session is almost finished and I thank everyone.

At the end of the session Violet said: "Today was different, less relaxing and peaceful than the first time!" In fact, we worked a lot on her fear. She was incredibly good at letting go of a lot of things in just one session.

Feedback:
Violet's mother would first like to share her appreciation regarding the last session. She likes the fact that I didn't push Violet to give up the doll. Earlier, a psychologist tried to force her to take away the doll, and as a result Violet shut down completely and stopped cooperating.

She told me that her daughter was doing very well. Violet was interacting more during family conversation, and taking part with the right timing and topic of the conversation. She also said she was looking more present and happier every day.

Third Session (November)
Before we began the session I asked Violet and her mother what the priority was today, Violet said that she was feeling tired. She was also excited to have a session.

Consuelo Cassotti B.S.

The session starts. Violet says: "I would like to be more present, like I was in the last period."

I pick up that she isn't afraid of growing up anymore. She is looking to be more engaged socially; she is very open to having conversations with other people, and I see an image of her talking, very relaxed and happy.

Violet explains: "When I have conversations with other people, I like to have Naruto with me because it is like a boy friend, a bodyguard; I feel safe!"

I feel that at this time it is a good idea to accept this need of Violet's. I ask her Future self to show up, but I feel some rigidity. It will happen when it is the right time, but not today.

I tell her soul: "You can be whoever you want to be." The way that she is looking at me, soul to soul, shows that this time, she is starting to believe it. She is thinking that it is possible!

I feel her head is now more organized and clear. We work on her belly, her colon and her sexual organs: second and first chakras. She asks her Angels directly, to work on something that she is worried about. I cannot say what it is because she allows me to hear but I do not know specifically what she is asking, and she doesn't explain to me. (I feel that she isn't comfortable with me knowing about it and I respect her privacy.)

They work on her head and her heart, to clear and take care of what she asked for. They work on her spine and her nervous system, to help her to relax more. For some reason the Angels work at different times on her ears, it is something about listening. It could be metaphoric; listen to yourself, or listen to others. Then they work on the other senses, to clear all of them.

(Regular conversation) Violet yawns...she says: "I am tired." She has released some exhaustion that she was holding for a period.

I help her to move her legs with some Polarity movements. This helps to release some tension, and she is feeling better. The session is over. I thank everyone.

Violet had a great holiday. She managed the excitement of Thanksgiving very well. According with her mother, we planned to wait to see if she can wait until January to have another session.

⁊ ⁌

Fourth Session (January)

When Violet arrived, I delete have sensed that she was in great need of a session.

We work on her nervous system. The reason why they start in this specific place is because of her excitement. Violet is very excited to be here today and she was waiting for this moment, and preparing herself for this appointment for days. My impression is right.

(Regular conversation) Her mother said: "Yes it is true, she began asking 10 days ago when would we come for her session."
I suggest that next time we don't leave so much space between one session and the next. We have been trying to leave 7 weeks between sessions, but it is probably too long too wait at this time. Her mother says: "She has been good, but she started to have some moments of anxiety two or three days ago..." I can see some excitement that affects her bowel movements.

We work on something belonging to her childhood. She was 6 or 7 years old, and it is something that might appear silly to others, but at the time it was important to her. Today, this is something

Consuelo Cassotti B.S.

that she could easily work through on her own because she is more mature.

I see people laughing and making fun of her.

(Regular conversation) Her mother says: "This week, Violet was talking about this."

I can see that at the time, she was expressing something that others didn't see. Something that she could perceive but because they could not, they made fun of her. This created in her some defense that remained. She began to shut down to what she was seeing and feeling, she didn't feel comfortable being in touch with this side of herself. I don't know what she was seeing, maybe angels or fairies, but she wasn't afraid because they were her friends. However, because others made fun of her, she stopped believing that she could see them. I feel that this is the primary reason why she is using a doll like Naruto as a friend, because she renounced the notion of having the other "invisible" friends.
They work on her ovaries, as though she is having some problem.

(Regular conversation) Her mother explains: "She is having some problems with her period, the doctor is changing some medications because she is having a heavy menstrual period."

Her body is fully covered with butterflies! We work on her spine, her full body; they regenerate her.
I look at Violet's mother, because I have information from my Spirit Guides that includes her too:
(Regular conversation) I needed to explain the information that I was receiving: "They are telling me that Violet is here, in

this family because of you. You decided some time ago about the possibility of having a child with some disabilities. I am talking about the fact that your soul gave permission to receive into your life, a child like Violet. You had thought that you would be able to manage someone like her. They are telling me that you are a person without judgment and very open to diversity. They are telling me that this is one of your powerful skills. You allowed yourself to have her. When they asked, you answered: Yes. Sometimes the request is made during the night, and subconsciously we decide.

Violet's mother looked at me and said: "I remember exactly when this happened! I was a teenager, like sixteen years old. I went to visit a place with children with special needs. During this visit I thought: "If I would have a child like this, I would manage."

I added: "Because of this, Violet arrived."

Violet shows me a place where she doesn't feel different or derided. It looks like a dreamland, a place where she can be a princess and be happy. I don't understand if it is her desire or another dimension where she goes sometimes. She is also telling me that lately she has had many exciting situations, all very positive, but she is feeling exhausted. A lot is going on.

To receive this session today helps her to release the tension. Sometimes she needs this, some help to reset her mind. It arrives to me that she might enjoy some breath work or some yoga exercises where she can learn breathing techniques. I see her sit and breathe. We work on her breathing, her diaphragm.

She feels very well and the session is done. I thank everyone.

Feedback:

Violet's was feeling well and more involved in activities where she can express herself. Her mother told me that at the appointment with the psychologist something very interesting happened. Violet explained why she carried Naruto with her. She said that she recognized her need to feel safe and that he is only a doll. The psychologist's "jaw dropped." She was surprised to hear such a logical and mature explanation from Violet.

৵৽

Sixth Session (March)
Violet was fine, she didn't have a particular request.

We experience some moments of adjustment with the energy. I notice that she is "energetically" separated, and it looks like the left side and the right side were divided. I would not be surprised if she has been feeling tired, in particular if her legs felt heavy. The left leg looks like it has lower energy.

(Regular conversation) I share this information with Violet's mother and she confirms the week before her daughter was having some problems in this leg.

Because the left side is related to our intuition, I feel that Violet's difficulty with her leg has something to do with the work she is undertaking in this area. Because her attempts to be more open to the positive voices of her intuition are complicated by the negative voices of her schizophrenia, this is much more of a challenge. I believe the physical symptoms are a confirmation of her need to be more confident in her intuition, which she is indeed working on.

I talk to Violet's soul: "Remember how beautiful and good you are. Remember that you can be more grown up. It is possible."

She answers me: "Sometimes I am afraid of the dark, not the dark like a room without a light, but the dark as a place or situation that she sees as dark, because it is unknown." I explain to her: "You can be stronger than this dark. You can always turn on the light that you have inside of yourself. Because of your beautiful bright light, you are always safe and in condition to manage any kind of darkness." For the moment then, she is very peaceful and calm. What she just expressed, is the only anxiety that she is having.

She tells me: "Sometimes I am very angry, because some people are very mean." I feel that in her mind, her world, she doesn't understand how and why people aren't nice to each other. It doesn't make any sense to her. It's like it is impossible for her to figure out how that can be.

(Regular conversation) Violet says: "I would like to work on "letting go of some things."

They work on her emotions: to be afraid or feel inferior. We want to help her to build more self esteem, and the possibility to stand up for what she thinks or likes. We work on her wings. The more she can move her wings and feel them, the sooner she can "fly."
We also work on releasing some toxins. It looks like she is eating something different than usual.

(Regular conversation) I ask Violet: "How are you doing?" She says: "I am feeling more active than I normally do during our sessions." I explain to her: "Today we are charging you more than usual."

Consuelo Cassotti B.S.

It arrives to me to use some tuning forks, one specifically for releasing fear, and another to ground her more. I play them. They harmonize all the work done.

(Regular conversation) Violet asks: "Mom, what can we do for lunch?"

I smile, she is so charged and relaxed that she is hungry. The session is over. I thank everyone.

Violet's update: She has a new friend. A nice and sweet boy, like her. They are starting to spend some time together, going to the theater, and some activities at school. They are like best friends or maybe a little more. She is so happy to spend some time with him.

ৰেঞ্জ

Seventh Session (April)
Violet was smiling, it appeared that she has enjoyed this moment every time.

The session starts. Today she is different, and she is lighter. It looks like she is surrounded by different beings, lighter with higher vibrations.

She tells me: "I am having a hard time leaving the past behind."

I feel her way of thinking, of perceiving... she is afraid to let go of thoughts, ideas, objects related to the past, because she has the impression that if she does, she can lose the past forever.

I feel that she thinks if she doesn't keep remembering the past, she cannot control the full picture anymore; she can lose the reference points.

For some reason, she tells me: "I feel very related to my sister, more than usual." She explains: " I want to become more of an adult." I feel that this idea is a link to her sister.

(Regular conversation) Violet's mother explained to me that the other daughter, a student at the university, arrived at home for Easter and she surprised everybody by announcing that she has a job. Evidently, this event affected Violet. She started to desire to be more grown up, because her sister is. I feel that something has clicked inside her and we are going to see more positive changes.

We work on her nervous system and on her brain. We clear unnecessary, past thoughts from the mind. I use this powerful moment: that she wants to grow up. I begin to explain what it can mean to be grown up. I tell her: "You can like or dislike some people or situations, and express this, nicely. You don't need to be afraid to offend people when you express your opinion. It is part of becoming an adult."

This time, she is listening. I feel that we have planted a seed that will grow. Normally she says that she is afraid to say "no" to people, because she doesn't want to offend them, but today she is handling this conversation without objections.

I see some butterflies cover her body, and she is happier and lighter! She asks me: "Can you make me more balanced?" The pictures that she sends me are about the way that she walks. She is afraid to fall. She moves in a way that she feels unbalanced. We work on this request.

She tells me: "I have had this feeling from an early age."

(Regular conversation) I ask her mother if she had any problem with walking or learning to walk. Her mother explains that

she had required therapy from the beginning. When she was 15 months old, she had a hip problem. For a long period, she was always in therapy.

Violet's soul tells me: "I had a bad experience when I was little." She probably fell, and she was so afraid that she still has the feeling of fear, and so she isn't completely confident in the way she walks. We clear these emotions and help her to be more balanced.
The session is over. I thank everyone.

ॐ∽

Eighth Session (May)

Violet was happy, she was very busy every day with a lot of activities. She was eager to work.

Immediately they start to work on many places at the same time. It looks like she is being helped to release a lot of tension, toxins and thoughts. Now I hold her head, as they asked me to help her with my hands to facilitate some releasing with some basic craniosacral positions. She is very sensitive to any changes to the environment...she can feel the shifts that are happening during this period on the Planet.

I ask my Beings if there is any way to shield her, to create a "filter" so she can be more balanced. They answer: "Yes and no. Because if they put too many filters in place, she will not feel many other good things, like good emotions." They work on her to create the filter. She is happy to have something that will help her to manage her every day incidents better. They work on cleaning and recharging the prana tube. They remove some yeast from her skin, and this period could be a time when the yeast affects her more than usual.

(Regular Conversation) Violet's mother tells me that her daughter had a sandwich today, but otherwise she is doing well with her diet.

We work on her nervous system, her third eye, and her way of expressing herself; her throat.

They tell me that Violet could have some problems for 2 or 3 months. She will have some difficulty until September. After September, she can begin to cut down on the dosage of her medications (of course always under doctor's supervision.)

I gave her mother this information in a regular conversation.

Violet showed me her wings. She looks at me very proudly, and she moves her wings like she can fly! This is very positive, because it means that she is becoming more confident.

I check to see if she is still worried about expressing herself, and also about her concern over disagreement with others. Happily, I find that she doesn't have the same feeling. She can express herself more confidently. What she has now, is the caring. She cares about others, but is not afraid to offend them anymore. It looks like she is growing more each time. She can manage more easily.

(Regular conversation) Her mother confirmed what I was feeling and expressing about Violet.

I play my crystal bowls to harmonize the work done. The session is finished and I thank everyone.

Violet's update: Her mother tells me that Violet doesn't complain anymore about chores and other things. She is acting more like a mature person.

෴

Consuelo Cassotti B.S.

Ninth Session (July)

Before we began the session, I noticed that Violet had substituted the doll Naruto, with a stuffed camel. This is just a toy though, and perhaps she doesn't need a stuffed *friend* any more.

We start to work on her mind, to clear some thoughts and some emotions. From what I see, I have the impression that today it is more about cleaning, recharging and balancing. We work on her breathing, because it looks like she has some problem, perhaps a cold.

Violet cannot stay around people who are very judgmental. This shows up today at different times.

They create an energy "bridge" between the right side and the left of her brain, and they say: "She is ready, she can manage this connection now." It looks like she could not manage this before, but now she is ready. I see that she is using more filters when she listens to a conversation. She knows what is important to hear and what isn't. She has more discernment.

I use some tuning forks and my rose quartz and amethyst crystal bowl. I see something come out of her body. It looks like her DNA is releasing/changing.

(Regular conversation) I explain to Violet's mother about what I have just seen, and I add: "Let me know if you see any positive change in the next weeks."

The session is over. I thank everyone.

Violet is coming for sessions every 3 to 4 months now. She is gradually leaving the twelve-year-old girl behavior behind her, without a second thought. It is also nice to see that the expression of her face is changing; she looks more like an adult. She acts more like a mature adolescent. She is taking a nice path, where she is finally less afraid of expressing herself and enjoys her life more. It has been a long period now since she has had any bad thoughts or anxious moments. She is finally a butterfly!

The fact that, with her parents more involved in energy work for themselves, has helped Violet to have a more harmonic transition

I have the impression, that most of her schizophrenic problems were created because she can hear and see things that most others cannot. Her difficulty was to be confident enough to create a filter that gave her more discernment.

*Update:
In August, Violet began to have strong seizures. On one such incident, while her parents were away, Violet was at home and she was apparently walking down the stairs when she began to have a seizure and fell, breaking her ankle. She lay there on the floor until her parents arrived home, shortly after. She was not afraid, but exercised the patience and logic of a mature young lady, knowing that her mother was due to arrive home shortly. This kind of composure was not something that Violet could have maintained just one year earlier.

When her mother informed me of what had happened, I recalled the occasion during my session, in May, with Violet, as they told me that she "could begin to have some problems for a few months" because of the shift in the energies. I felt then as I certainly do now, that this was exactly what

Consuelo Cassotti B.S.

they were referring to. I feel that this is something that is very important for people who experience seizures to be aware of, that the changing energetic vibrations, though they represent a shift for the better, may at times bring with them a natural swing of the energetic pendulum, so to speak. Therefore in order to bring things into balance, they must first be forced slightly out of kilter in the opposite direction, before coming to rest in position. As in Violet's case, this nudge that created the energetic momentum for change, may be the actual cause of the seizure condition, and therefore a necessary but temporary condition. As for others with a seizure condition, I feel it is important and worthwhile to consider the implications of energetic work, and its bearing and value as a possible treatment for such conditions.

Chapter 4
The warrior of light trapped in his own emotions.

Everyone knows that teenagers have some difficulty expressing their emotions and saying what they want to say. If we look at the combination of low confidence and their high sensitivity to the environment, we can easily see why they struggle to figure out who they are and what their path is if they don't have the right help.

Most of the adolescents that I see are having a hard time talking to counselors or psychologists because of the stigma attached to visiting these professionals. The reason why my sessions are so successful with them is because they do not need to speak, and because of this they feel more comfortable and understood. I am able to pick up on their inner emotions immediately, and am guided as to the best way to help them. To my surprise, most look forward to coming to my sessions!

Sometimes my sessions are done in my healing room and other times I work by distance. Even though the results are the same, this is a distinct advantage for some children, since they needn't feel as though "they have to be fixed" or go through another intervention.

᷈᷉

Consuelo Cassotti B.S.

When I first met Stephen I noticed his poor posture, and his body language told me that he was having a hard time standing up for himself. It was difficult for him to make eye contact for very long and he had a sullen look and sadness about him. Stephen was tall and slim, and his mother explained to me that he had always had a difficult time expressing his emotions. He had suffered with asthma off and on throughout his life and seemed to always separate himself from the rest of the family. Thanks to his mother, he agreed to work with me.

First Session (February)
Stephen appeared open to receive the session.

The session starts. Immediately (and) we work to release some anger issues from his navel and I can see a volcano erupting. We work on his mind, clearing out some old thoughts and old belief systems that no longer serve him. He has a hard time relaxing completely, as his body is very tense. We work on the nervous system... and his joints and legs, because he is still growing. I cannot see his wings, I believe because it is too early. I cannot touch his heart. He is very private and he needs more time to trust me fully. Then, we work on his lungs, liver and stomach. I speak to his soul : "Remember who you are, you can be who you want to be"

I feel that I planted a seed and we will see what future sessions will do for him. I use some sound therapy and tuning forks to assist him. Finally, I felt some sadness leave his body! The beings that were surrounding him have very high energy. They were also very tall like him, and it looks like they were mostly angels. He starts to release a lot of stuff. I see a lot of pictures with faces ... too fast to pick up on any certain one, but this is a way for the mind to clear and become clean. I ask his soul another question: "Who do you want to be?" The look in his etheric eyes told me: "I don't know." I feel that he lacks passion in his life. I remind him: "You can be anyone you want!"

I have the impression that there is somebody around him who tends to put him down a lot.

(Regular Conversation) I ask him: " What is the difference between today and one year ago?" He explains: "My cousin moved in to our home and he is attending the same school as I am. I try to be nice to him because he had a very difficult childhood, but he makes me so mad sometimes."

We work on his anger and help him to release any emotions from this relationship. I could feel that he was less tense.

After 30 minutes or so the session is over. I thank everyone.

I feel I planted the seed and helped to awaken his soul. Only time will tell.

After our session I asked him if he felt anything. He answered me: "No" but I got the impression that he was accustomed to not expressing anything at all. I could see that his face had more color and he was not frowning so much. I could see a little smile on his face!

I later learned from Stephen's mother that this cousin had suffered a very difficult childhood; in fact John was adopted. John was very competitive and put Stephen down quite a bit. Stephen had overcome his childhood asthma but was starting to experience more episodes in the last

Consuelo Cassotti B.S.

year. Stephen lives with his mother, stepfather and autistic brother.

☙ ❧

Second Session (March)
Immediately after he arrived he said:" Hi, can you work on my breathing today?" I sensed he was having hard time breathing. He took off his tennis shoes, and to my delight jumped onto the massage table. The session began.

I feel some sadness, and a mix of emotions. I see through his eyes; watching his younger brother play with his step-father, and feeling a mix of jealousy and a sense of guilt toward his little brother... Stephen never experienced this type of interaction with his real father and part of him missed this kind of relationship.

(Regular conversation) I carefully express: "I see this picture and I feel these emotions..." Stephen's eyes welled up with tears. Stephen says: "We went to an amusement park a week ago..." and this is the trigger to help him to let go. I explain to him: "It is normal to have these feelings. The little child inside of you misses his dad."

I feel his love for his little brother Alex, but also some difficulty with accepting some other (not-so-loving) emotions toward him.
We work on this very gently and slowly. Stephen finally starts to open up his heart with me. We work on the scarring in his heart. In the meantime I talk to his inner child, reassuring him that he is loved by his family. The more we work on his heart, the more I see it is expanding, full of energy and love! It is a beautiful vision. He is finally opening himself up to receive more love.

(Sometimes breathing problems are related to the emotions of the heart, like love and sadness.)

I see one being holding Stephen's ankles, he needs to be more grounded. Another being is working on his shoulders. I can barely see his wings, but they look more like butterfly wings; very colorful and fragile, versus angel wings. I never saw wings like this before.

His anger for his cousin John shows up again. We clear the emotional cord connecting them.

We finish balancing and integrating the work we did.

The session is over. I thank everyone.

We didn't have time to discuss what happened, he seemed to be in hurry to leave. I contacted his mother a few days later to get some feed back about his breathing and emotions. I believed that he went very deep during the session, and typically when someone goes very deep the physical symptoms can become exacerbated until they are totally cleared.

His mother answered me: "Stephen is off school today. He can only handle a few hours at school each day because his breathing and his chest feel stiff." This did not surprise me since it takes time to release old emotions completely. It was part of the healing process.

Working with energy healing requires the proper timing, to change and handle the shifts in the energy. Sometimes it can happen in a few minutes, other times it is so deep that it requires more than one session. This was obviously a big shift for Stephen but I was encouraged to see that he was willing to start to heal himself.

Consuelo Cassotti B.S.

I had emailed Stephen's mother, regarding my intuitive impression about the impact his cousin John was having on Stephen's self esteem. In fact, I had noticed that John was coming up in every session. I thought it would be a good idea to do a distance session to both of them at the same time, since they were related emotionally. I wanted to help them both be more balanced and have more harmony in their relationship. Of course, I would need to ask permission to both souls, and if the answer was yes I could teach Stephen to set more boundaries with John.

ॐ•ॐ

Third Session–given by distance to Stephen and his cousin, John.

(Before to start the session, I asked John's soul the permission to work on him, he gave to me a permission).

They have very different energies. John's energy is strong and persistent; Stephen's energy is more gentle and light. I began by working on their hearts. I clear both hearts at the same time, to set things in order. I clear the emotional cord between them, and I ask that they be connected with love, nothing else. We work on John... his skin is very itchy, his cells are so full of anger. It is a very strong anger energy. He is angry most of the time, and has a hard time letting go of this energy because anger is something that he knows well and is comfortable with. For him, being in this energy means to be in his safe place, something that he is used to. We began cleaning this emotion and started sending him unconditional love and light. He became upset with me. He was so addicted to this angry energy that he didn't like that I was trying to help him. He began to calm down. I could see then, that when John comes close to Stephen, he cannot breathe and he feels suffocated. He cannot think, act or be himself freely. I see that this connection needs to be more neutral. One angel talks to John and explains to him that what he does and thinks affects not only himself, but also those around him. John listens to the angel, and this is a good sign.

Stephen looks tired because he is supporting his cousin; he gives up too much of his own energy. Next, the same angel talks to Stephen and explains to him how to be in a healthier relationship with John and not be affected by him. This angel carries a very high energy.

These 2 boys are very different, like black and white. There is a sort of competition going on between them. John instigates this competition and knows that Stephen will not stand up for himself. We send more unconditional love so that they both feel complete. John then yells at me, stating that he didn't like what we are doing (probably because he never felt unconditional love before.) Again, John has begun to relax, and then finally allowed himself to receive love. John is very sharp and likes to push peoples' buttons. He likes to get negative reactions from people. He has suffered a lot of trauma, and battles the shadows. Stephen hasn't suffered with such deep trauma and is trying to solve his issues. John seems to be stuck in his "deep mud" of trauma. Stephen appears to be breathing better. He yawns (as a sign of releasing), good! The session is over. I thank everyone.

After this session, Stephen's mother understood better the fragile balance between her son and her nephew.

Fourth Session (June)

Stephen's mother was concerned that he did not finish the school year with good grades and I was feeling that she doubted her son's future. She was afraid that he would end up like his biological father, a person without goals and little success. When Stephen arrived for his session he agreed to work with me on his focus and his memory.

I start the session. We immediately begin working on his mind to clear thoughts that were no longer necessary, and to make more space for knowledge. I ask his spirit guides to increase his memory, and they told me that it was possible to increase it by 15%. They work on Stephen's head. I notice that they took wires from different parts of his head and restored them energetically, to help with the flow. It looks like a computer or electric panel with golden wires. They create a bridge between the left and the right side of the brain, to more fully integrate his knowledge.

They say that Stephen is a "warrior of light," and that he needs to remember who he is. Everywhere he goes he takes light with him and his vibration affects others in a very positive way. As a "warrior of light" he is very supported by his brothers (both currently incarnated and not). I am watching them, and they look very similar to Stephen; like angels, tall and thin with incredibly sweet and shy expressions in their eyes.

They work on his nervous system to facilitate the flow in the body. Stephen is still growing and his body is having a hard time keeping up with the rapid changes in all his physical parts. They work on his legs, joints, muscles and nerves. Part of this session, looks more like a maintenance session, or a session to help him be more balanced. (Not every session goes so deep emotionally). The session is over. I thank everyone.

Finally, his cousin John didn't show up this time and Stephen seemed more balanced about this relationship.

∂∘◌

Since working on Stephen I have found other children/teenagers named by their spirit guides and angels as "warriors of light." They look physically and energetically very similar. They are here to ground a particular energy on the planet and they are beacons of light. I can still recall the image of them that was shared with me, and how their mere presence helps those around them, because of their energy. I believe they belong to the same grid, a group of souls with a similar mission. Even when they are not so conscious about their mission, they are effective and they are all connected. I am pretty sure that when they go to sleep they share information with their brothers.

∂∘◌

Fifth Session (July)

Stephen looked more serene and calm than when I first met him. His breathing was normal. He did open up and share with me that he was tired of seeing himself with little focus and memory. He complained about his difficulty concentrating at school and focusing in conversation. He also told me that he had a hard time remembering what he ate for breakfast that day. He wished he was the same person he felt like 2 years earlier, when he had good grades at school and he felt his life was more successful. He also said that at times he felt a pressure on the top or front of his head after the last session. (His mother reported that his diet was much better 2 years ago and she could sense a decline since he stopped eating the better way.)

Consuelo Cassotti B.S.

We begin the session with the desire to increase his brain skills and his ability to concentrate. A tall, high energy being arrives and focuses on the top of Stephen's head. I can see a rectangular gray metal plate situated in the front of Stephens's head (energetically speaking of course, in this 3D world it doesn't exist) and the being explained to me that it was a vow that he took with him into this life.

For some reason, Stephen agreed to live this life with this implant or energetic block, for the purpose of being less intelligent. I have the impression that in a past life he was a very brilliant scientist or inventor, and he created something that was used improperly and caused death. He felt so guilty and ashamed of what had happened that he created this contract in order to sabotage himself in this current lifetime. He was too afraid to make a similar mistake. The beings told me that Stephen placed it there, but now that he has asked for help, we could remove most of the block. I am instructed to do it slowly, and during the course of the session. In the meantime, we work on other parts of his body...helping his nervous system, his legs, and we clear away some toxins. We also work on recharging his body. I notice that Stephen's implant is becoming very small and they tell me that they need 10 minutes more.

(Regular conversation) Stephen says: "I am feeling less pressure in my head and my scalp is ticklish."
I reply: "A few minutes more and the session will be over."

In fact after some minutes, the session is over. I thank everyone.

After the session, I realized that Stephen and John had made a deal before coming into this lifetime. Stephen prob-

84

ably asked his cousin to treat him badly and beat him down prior to incarnating into this lifetime, as part of this contract.

In some way, John was giving Stephen such a hard time because it was part of the plan. Unconsciously, John did this as an act of love.

Sixth Session (August)

Stephen came for another session. I was so amazed to see him look so much better (I am not sure if his mother noticed.) His face was glowing, his energy was more expansive, and his eyes were very deep and very clearly intense!

Just as I had told his mother back in the spring, he would be feeling better by the summer. Stephen confirmed that he was feeling more like he did 2 years ago, through doing well at school and being full of energy. He paid more attention to detail and was more focused. His mind was clear. Stephen jumped onto the table, very open and relaxed, without any resistance.

I open the session and he is deeply relaxed, which never happened before. His Spirit Guides and mine tell me that now he can pursue everything he wants!

The decision is made. Stephen decided to be smarter, without fear of the past. I am so happy to witness the moment, it is like a caterpillar that becomes a butterfly. His wings are more like angel wings now, stronger.

This year at school he will have a wonderful time, he will attract only positive people/situations. They tell me that now, part of him knows his "mission" and he will understand more as time goes by, because he became stronger and he is free of the blocks that he had in the past years. His life is going to be more positive and balanced because of his "change of mind." His Future Self then shows up, and I can see him being an IT teacher or training consultant. He is happy and very confident.

We clean some parasites/infections from his body.

We remove some stress, related to the sports that he is participating in and from summer classes.

We work on various parts of his body; nervous system, lungs... Everything seems to be better. The session is over. I thank everyone.

Finished the session, I told him to honor the fact that he was open enough to make the shift. Everything happened because he wanted it. I have only helped him to do it.

He needed to recognize his will to be more open and to face his difficulties.

I am very happy for him!

After Stephen left, I wrote an email to his mother, wherein I said that from this moment, I was sure that Stephen would have a brighter future. I reminded her that we always have opportunities to change our destiny and fulfill our dreams ... I said: "Give him a chance and you will be surprised!"

*Update: the following year was Stephen's last year of high school. His grades were so high that he was accepted into a local college. Stephen came back to see me a few times for maintenance sessions, due to typical high school stressors.

He hasn't experienced any more asthma symptoms either. At the end of the school year he got a great full-time summer job, and did well. His mother and stepfather were so proud of him because he showed them how he could focus and be strong enough to manage the job. He even started to date a nice girl and life was flowing nicely for him.

He is in college now, and working toward following his true path; the path that his future self showed him. I know that this "warrior of light" has spread his wings and is going to fly!

Chapter 5
The girl that never slept until she discovered dreams

The first time that Lisa and her mother came to my healing room, it was like a tornado was going through my place. She was running and yelling without stopping. Lisa was eight years old and she could not sit still for more than one minute. It didn't surprise me that her mother was talking in a fast and high tone, like a person with some anxiety.

Lisa was very skinny and very hyperactive. She could not stop, and was always in motion. Her mother told me that she was autistic, but her visual contact was good and she was very coordinated. She spoke as though she was younger, in comparison to other children her age. I didn't feel as though she was like the other autistic children that I had worked with before. I had a feeling that she was different.

Lisa's mother told me that she was having a hard time at school and at home. She was constantly in motion, jumping on the furniture, never resting. She would sleep only briefly during the night, and this was affecting the "regular life" of her parents, who had to take shifts at night to guard Lisa while she was awake.

Consuelo Cassotti B.S.

First Session (June)

I asked Lisa to sit down, and she had a hard time staying in the chair. I asked her mother to give her some coloring books so that she could color. It seemed (to) work.

The session starts. I am feeling her high vibration, her energy is strong and fast. We want to help her be more grounded and to calm down a little. She sit still and allows everyone to work on her. We work on her nervous system, and also her joints and muscles. They work on her brain, to slow down the energy. She started to be calmer.

I talk to her, and ask her to be more calm and present. I tell her that her parents love her and they are looking for a way to communicate with her. She is surprised that I can talk to her, but she is not interested in changing her way of being or her life. She said to me: "I love the life that I have! My parents are always so nice, and they want always to please me. I can ask them for anything I want, and they do it! Why do I need to change?!"

She shows me her wings, she knows how to use them. I am feeling that she is having a hard time being in her body because she is carrying a very high vibration (like an angels' vibration), and her body is having a hard time adjusting completely. She begins walking around. She stops communicating with me, but my beings are keeping up with her, and they continue to work on her as she moves.

They align her back and her shoulders... her posture. She comes back to the chair, but then decides to sit on the floor. We work on the top of her head and in many other parts. We clear her "prana tube", liver, and pancreas. They give her a lot of liquid. It looks like she is dehydrated.

(Regular conversation) I suggest to her mother that she have her drink more water than pop or sodas. She needs good water.

It seems enough for today. The session is over. I thank every-one.

After the session I have decided to write an email to her mother. I want to explain to her how important it is to set some rules and boundaries with Lisa. Lisa's life is happy, but her parents are paying the price. It doesn't seem fair. This family needs to find more balance. Lisa needs some challenges and rules to help her to mature. I suggest they start with little steps, but be consistent. Without rules she will be a selfish teen-ager, who will create trouble. Good rules and boundaries are important in shaping a child's personality.

I remember once during a session with another child, a female arrived and began to yell and admonish the young boy who was receiving a session from me. I was astonished! I had never seen this before. I asked to understand more about this. The explanation I was given was about how it is important that a child play as a child, with some rules, and parents need to be consistent and balanced in their role. In this case this boy dictated his parents life. His mother was passive with low self-esteem, and his father preferred to travel rather than face the situation. The boy was so upset because they didn't provide any strict rules, and he felt that they didn't care about him.

Consuelo Cassotti B.S.

Second Session (given by distance, July)

A month later, Lisa's mother could not bring her daughter to the next appointment so we decided to do a distance session. Lisa's mother said that she noticed some improvement in her daughter. She was using more vocabulary, but she was still jumping on the furniture.

We work immediately to calm her down. She yells at us: "It isn't fair!" I feel that her body is in pain and she doesn't like being so present in this painful body. My Spirit Guides explain to me that tonight at 10:00 PM she will calm down completely. It looks like she is angry about something. At this moment Lisa doesn't talk to me, she doesn't want to share anything.

We work on her legs, to help her be more grounded. I feel the pain in her body, I have some difficulty understanding why she has this problem. I tell her that everything is fine and that sometimes it can be hard to be fully present in the body, if you didn't have this habit before. You feel more deeply what you have in your life, but this is part of the deal. To be present in your body, means also that it is possible to do more interesting things. I tell her that she is loved by her parents, and that she can be more like a "grown up" girl. She looks at me and says: "I like it!"

I tell her that if she wants to be in charge of her life, she needs to be more present, needs to be more in her body, and to be more focused everyday. To reach this goal, she also needs to be nice to her body; sleep some hours, rest a little sometimes, give herself time to recharge her batteries. If she does this, she can enjoy her life more. She looks at me, very focused in what I am saying to her. She is listening!

She really likes the idea: "to be more in charge," she repeats these words one more time. She likes the way they sound, and she likes what it means. She explains to me that being more present in her body isn't so much fun. I explain to her how cool it is to get a massage from her mom, how nice it is to play with other children, to taste good food...you can really taste more.

At this same time, I can feel some imbalance in our conversation....I finally understand the reason why her body is in pain! My beings tell me that she is eating too much sugar. It is very important to reduce her intake of sugar. She has too much sugar in her system and this isn't good at all.

Next they work on balancing the chakras. They are willing to help her to grow up a little more, emotionally and mentally. She is helped to become a little more mature. Her way of thinking, acting, everything appropriate to her age level is changing. They increase the size of each of the chakras. First they increase them by 3%. The first chakra is about being more present and more grounded. They are going to increase this chakra a little more before the session is finished. They help harmonize all the chakras and any work done in this session.

I explain to Lisa how nice it would be if she would start to slow down a little bit, and be calmer and happy, so that she can enjoy the company of her parents and brother more.

The session is over. I thank everyone.

I suggested to the parent: "For the next session, we need to figure out something that she likes to do, but is struggling with. Then I can push her to be more present and focus on reaching this goal. Also, it is very important to decrease her intake of sugar."

Sometimes distance sessions are more efficient, because I don't need to deal with the additional job of handling the child's behavior in my room. Normally I do the distance sessions during their sleep time, when the person is more receptive. In Lisa's case, because she never sleeps more than 3 to 4 hours at night, I did the session when I felt the time was right.

Lisa's mother told me that her daughter showed some independence, she didn't want to go to sleep with her mother like she usually did, but instead she stayed alone. She also displayed other mature behaviors during her daily routine. Her mother said: "I am happy for her, but I am missing my baby." I have noticed that some parents with a challenged child have some difficulty letting the child grow up. In their mind, they want to protect him/her so badly, that it becomes a disadvantage to the child.

Third Session (given by distance, August)

The day the third session was scheduled, Lisa had a fever and she could not come. I asked my Spirit Guides if it was possible to give her a session. I wanted to help her feel better, and I didn't want to lose the effect of the previous sessions. In the beginning of the work, I prefer there not be too much time between sessions.

To begin, we work on bringing down her fever. We use blue electric color to cool it. They tell me that we cannot do anything until the fever is gone. Because of this we wait several minutes, in order to give the body time to adjust.

We work to increase her immune system, by 20%. They also work on her blood system; red and white cells, and platelets. The tell me that there is some imbalance; she has more white cells than red. Of course, it is just at this present moment. I ask if there is any mercury or yeast that needs to be removed today. They said that she has them and that we can partially clear them, perhaps 15%. They do this very slowly during the entire session. If she becomes a little nauseated it is because of this work. They work on her first chakra. A lot of yellow powder comes out of her vagina, and it looks like yeast is also coming out. If she has been experiencing some itching lately it is because of some candida infection,

Lisa looks at me with an expression of relief on her face. She tells me that she is doing better, and that she feels more balanced. She looks very surprised to feel better.

The work on the yeast is not yet finished and she is continuing to release yellow powder. We check the joints and the nervous system. I explain to her again how it is important to be present in her body, so she can speak better and be more easily understood by other people.

(Regular conversation) I explained to Lisa's mother that Lisa's future self is showing up. Because of this I told her not to be surprised if her daughter starts to mature faster during the coming months.

In fact, I see an adolescent of 14 or 15 years old, very confident about herself, naked. She loves her body and she likes to be wild and free. She looks very independent and in charge of her life, and she likes this.

We work on her digestive system. They say that she needs more good fat in her food.

Consuelo Cassotti B.S.

(Regular conversation) I told her mother that it would be nice if she added some extra virgin olive oil to Lisa's diet. Also, Omega 3 would be good. The walls of Lisa's stomach are in need of some good oil. Just a spoonful a day, in her regular food would suffice.

We check her ears, and they are a little inflamed, especially the right ear. An angel is working on her ears. He has very sweet energy. We work on the spine. She needs some stretching. It is important for removing the pain in the joints, and so the nervous system can be more relaxed.

I see some ankle bracelets on Lisa's ankles. I get the impression that they belong to a past life. These bracelets don't have a chain, but she wasn't able to be completely free. Today we release this memory. I am sure that we are going to see a better way to walk.

We oxygenated her skin, in particular the torso. We work on her breathing too. I notice that we are increasing the oxygen and I like this because I believe it will help her to think and speak better. I ask if we need to work on the liver and they say that they already did. Lisa shows me her wings. She is receiving an activation from the angels. Her wings are beautiful and big.

(Regular conversation) I told her mother not to be surprised if she starts to be more independent.

They work on her mouth, neck, and head. It looks like they are adjusting the electric lines; the energetic connection between speech and the brain. I can see different colors around her and her bodies. Because of this I ask the spiritual, mental, emotional and physical bodies to join together. I ask Lisa to forgive herself and all her parts. She seems very happy about this work, and we harmonize all the work done.

Because I see that she is very open to listening, I tell her that it is better if she sleeps more each night because then she will have less physical problems, like fever and fatigue. I ask her to try to sleep for 7 to 8 hours every night. I tell her to try it for 10 days and see how much better she feels. She said: "I can try it for a week." It isn't a very big yes, but at least we will see if she is willing to try.

(Regular conversation) I explain to Lisa's mother that Lisa will take several days to digest this session. She will be tired and sleepy for one or two days.

The session is over. I thank everyone.

It was a very deep session and I was surprised to see a young girl have such a session. This confirmed for me that she comes from a very high energy group of souls. It is the reason why she can handle a deep session so well.

Ten days later, I received an envelope with a check from Lisa's mother. Included was a note from Lisa's mother: "Thank you Consuelo for the incredible session... the fever went down. You were right, she did exactly what she had promised; every night she has slept 8 hours, for one week as you said. The 8th night she decided to have a party in her room at 2 am, and she never slept 8 hours again. We hope that she will come to understand how good it is to sleep more regularly. At school she is doing better. Her language is improving and her behavior too, when she has slept enough."

ॐ∽

Consuelo Cassotti B.S.

Between the session in August and the other at the end of September, I gave a short distance session to reinforce her sleeping behavior. I contacted her to emphasize the difference between when she was sleeping all night and when she wasn't, and how the activities became more difficult and challenging when she wasn't sleeping. She was listening. I had the impression that she also noticed the difference, and she was starting to realize how much better things were when she slept longer.

A few days after this short session, Lisa decided to sleep every night for 7 to 8 hours. Her mother told me that every night before she went to sleep, Lisa told her parents: "Night, night" and she went to sleep. She didn't need somebody to tell her to go to sleep.

∾∾

Fourth Session (given by distance, September)
Because of the good results from the distance sessions and the busy schedule of Lisa's mother, we decided to do the next session by distance. Her mother informed me that Lisa was coughing and that she had a fever.

Lisa is waving at me, she looks happy. I ask her how she is doing and she answers me: "Fine!"

We work on her cough. I can see mucus in her throat and in her heart. We clear some of this mucus to help her feel better. It looks like Light beings are helping her to release some toxins, and she really likes it.

They work on her legs, stretching and energizing them. They want to help her to be more flexible. I see some rings around her ankles. Lisa tells me that she created these rings, so that she can be more present in her body. She says: "This is my way to do it and I like it!"

We help her to breath more. We work on the diaphragm, because she needs more oxygen. We also work on her nervous system. She looks very relaxed. Lisa says: "I want to be a big girl!"

I ask her "How's school?" She answers: "School is ok. There are two boys that bother me." She sends me a picture of them: "One is big, with a round shaped body, and another is smaller." I feel that these two boys are not very nice to her and she is having some trouble being around them. She also shows me the picture of one teacher, she probably has blonde hair, and Lisa says: "I like her a lot."

Lisa tells me: "Mom is fine, she is doing fine." I have the impression that Lisa's mother is doing better, and she is resting more because Lisa is sleeping at night now.

I help her to readjust in her body. Her energy is big, and I can feel the expansion of her energy. I tell her: "Remember who you are."

I ask Lisa if I can clear some emotional cords from her, and she answers me: "Yes, go ahead." I call the Archangel Michael to do this job, and he does. She tells me that she thinks she wants to be a painter when she grows up. Something related to creativity, art and fashion.

I ask if she wants to say something to her mother, but she doesn't have anything in particular to say. I can feel her happiness, her excitement. These emotions are different from the first session. Now, it is as if everyday there is something nice to do, to learn....

I ask her: "How long do you want to be this way?" she answers: "Until I will be strong enough." I feel that she is in charge of what she is doing, more than the parents realize. She had needed these years to slow herself down, in order to adjust to this 3D energy.

I ask her: "Do you understand how important it is to sleep?" She answers: "Yes, it is interesting because when I sleep deep, I can dream."

(I now realize that she has never had an occasion to sleep deeply until now.)

The session is over. I thank everyone.

ॐॐ

Fifth session (October).

This time Lisa and her mother came to my office. Lisa was sitting in a chair busily reading. Her mother said that she was doing better.

The session starts, Lisa looks more balanced, but tired. I can see that she is in need to recharge.

(Regular conversation) I explain to her mother what I see and she confirms: "Lately, Lisa is running out of energy."

I feel that she is also absorbing a lot of emotions and tensions from the environment. The fact that her father is traveling and is absent for weeks, the possibility that the family will move to another state, most certainly creates some tensions at home.

We work on her stomach. We work on her speech. Lisa asks to be helped to speak clearly. She is still growing, and we stretch her legs and joints. I ask Lisa: "How's school?" she answers me: "Weeelll!" She explains: "I like to be at school because there is one girl that is very nice to me." I can see that this particular girl is helping Lisa, and she tells me that they play well together and un-

derstand each other. It doesn't matter how they communicate, they do.

(Regular conversation) I explain what I see/heard to her mother, and she confirms that she knows who the girl is, and she sees the harmony between them.

I reinforce how important it is to sleep well every night, and to be present in her body. I also ask her future self to show up and remind Lisa who she can be. She allows us to work on her heart. It is the first time that she has opened up completely!
I ask Lisa if she wants to say something to her mother and she says "No." She then shows me an image of her making a funny face while eating peas, and says: "I don't like them!"

(Regular conversation) I share this information with Lisa's mother. Laughing, she says: "Yes, she doesn't like peas."

The session is finished (in fact before I can say anything, and at the same time that I am closing the session, Lisa stands up and starts to run around...) I thank everyone.

At the end of the summer Lisa started in a new school. Her mother was concerned about the big change, but with some adjustment to her diet and my energy work, she seemed to be doing very well. At school, the teachers observed that Lisa was more curious about the activities, and she was more manageable. She can sit and play nice, and she was following directions.

Consuelo Cassotti B.S.

Sixth Session (given by distance, December)

Lisa's mother hasn't been able to take her at my office, but we don't want to leave too much time between on session and another. I gave her a distance session.

Lisa is very nervous, and has been having some tantrums. I see her acting like she doesn't want to do what others want. We work immediately on her brain, to slow down some energy. I call Archangel Michael, to clear the emotional cord from her father. I feel that this connection is unbalanced. I see other cords running back and forth, coming out of Lisa and connecting to other people. We are going to clear these cords, one at a time, throughout the session. Lisa is absorbing other people's emotions without knowing. The first emotional cord is related to her mother. We clear this connection; we want to leave only a neutral connection.

We also work on her body; joints, muscles, bones...I can see that her diet is better. Her body is much clearer. Her mind seems to work better.

She is opening her heart, but I feel that we need to be very cautious because she is very protective about her heart.

I see that her heart has boxes, and it looks like she has everybody she loves in a separate box. She doesn't have everybody together. She prefers to have separate relationships with every person she loves. I can hear her say: "I like this person because of this ... I love him because of that ... "

We want to help her have more harmony in her heart. We are knocking down some of the walls in her heart, so that she can love without pre-conceptions. We do this work very slowly and gently. She is doing very well. The way that she is communicating with me gives me the impression that her way of thinking is more mature.

Her future self seems only associated with a beautiful girl that loves herself, and is very self centered.

Lisa needs to be helped to realize that there is a future as a productive adult, not just a beautiful young lady.

I ask Lisa: "How is your mother?" She shows me picture of her house. There is too much clutter around the house. She doesn't like to stay in the house because it is too chaotic, and she feels nervous when she is at home. It seems that the house isn't a very balanced place for her, and in fact she prefers to be at school where everything is more organized and balanced.

We clear the second cord, which links her to her dad. She is missing her dad, and says: "I miss my daddy!"

Lisa points to her belly, and we work on her belly. She has more air in her colon than normal. It is an emotional issue related to her home. We are taking care of the third emotional cord, which links her to her brother. I can see a young boy close to her. We clear also the fourth cord, and it is connected to a couple of people, who are not so young. I have the feeling that they are grandpa and grandma.

We clear everything that is possible without creating any imbalance. Lisa is more relaxed than at the beginning of the session. She smiles at me. Now that she is free of any energy blocks and unbalanced connections, she is lighter and more relaxed.

The way that she refers to how people communicate with her makes me think that she can hear thoughts. Now a violet vortex surrounds her and ascended master Saint Germain shows up, and he is clearing her with this vortex energy, of all the dependencies that she was carrying. This is a beautiful moment ... Lisa had an incredibly deep session! The session is over. I thank everyone.

Consuelo Cassotti B.S.

After the session, I emailed the recorded session to Lisa's mother and I explained that it would be nice if she would start to create a dialogue with her daughter about: What you want to do in your future or when you are grown up? Talk about jobs, careers... goals.

I also suggested playing calm music at home and organizing her things in a way that she can find them easily. Set aside some time when everybody can stop and relax. At this time the house doesn't have any relaxing energy.

❧ ❧

Again, Lisa's case is yet another example of how important it is for the immediate family to be balanced, as well as the affected child.

Lisa's mother was going through a stressful period and Lisa described how it was affecting her.

Lisa's mother didn't have any sessions during the period that I worked with Lisa. She always thought that it was better to spend the money on her daughter. Parents typically spend what spare money they have on their children (and very unselfishly I might add), and are so riddled with guilt about the mere idea of spending any on themselves, that they do not realize how necessary it is for family balance. Sadly, without this balance it is difficult for the parents to work on their awareness too. By neglecting themselves and their part in the scheme of things, they lose some potential for more positive results with their child.

*Update: Lisa was changing rather quickly and this may have had an impact on her mother, and her mother's desire to keep her dependent on her. After several sessions

Lisa was becoming more independent, and no longer in need of a personal aide.

Lisa was finally eating healthier foods and putting on some weight for her height. Her speech was improving daily and the meltdowns were fewer and fewer. She was calmer and more cooperative. It appeared that Lisa wanted to be more mature for her age!

I am certain we could have seen more progress if the entire family had decided to work together. It appeared to me, that the results were enough to give the family the balance and quiet that they had needed for a long time, and too much change could have been too hard to handle.

I would have loved to see how far Lisa would have taken me, but at this moment I am probably the only person who desires this.

Chapter 6
The souls lost in the dark, finally reconnect with the light.

During the years, I have worked in different parts of the world with my distance sessions, and every time somebody asks me: "Can you work on this case or this problem?" my answer is: "Why not? Let me see what I can do for you."

I have noticed that when you believe that everything is possible, there is a big chance that the "magic" inside of the person will come out!

Like these case histories:

Once I worked on a young man named Renan from Brazil. He was suffering from depression for some years when his mother contacted me. She asked me to give him a distance session. At the time, he was 19 years old. He had stopped studying or doing anything that involved focus and energy. He was depressed.

Because Renan didn't speak English, we set a time where he was to just be relaxed on his couch, and open to receive this energy work. During the session I noticed that some parts of Renan were completely disconnected from him. He was always tired because of this. We worked to merge together his physical, mental, emotional and spiritual bodies. We worked very deeply on some memories from past lives. We awakened his soul, so that he could remember his "mission" in this lifetime.

Gradually, after this session he felt more energized and balanced. I never had the occasion to talk to him directly, but some weeks after his first session, his mother wrote me that her son felt more energized and balanced. He was waking up in the morning smiling; he started becoming more interested in going out and socializing.

Three months later, Renan's cousin Cristina (who was living in the USA and was my client for a long period) informed me that Renan had found a job and was doing well, but his mother wanted me to repeat another session to Renan. He was so full of energy that she thought Renan was in need of some help balancing his rest with his activity. He was so excited and full of energy that relatives and friends where asking him what happened to him. I have the impression that after I reached his soul and helped Renan to remember his mission in this life, he wanted to make up the "time lost." After a second session he seemed to be fine. A year later, Cristina said that Renan is having a nice life and is thinking about finishing his degree.

I am so amazed to see such incredible change in people in such a very short time! I think that it happens more easily when a person is ready and willing to face the challenges and the emotional blocks. Sometimes a traumatic memory or sense of guilt that is carried around from this life or a past life holds us down. Awakening the soul can be powerful when the person is willing to move on.

୭◦୶

Hearing a Different Voice

Recently in Australia, a client of mine asked me to work on her younger brother, Cody. She said that he was schizophrenic and she was hoping that I could reach his mind and help him to feel better.

At the beginning of my distance session, Cody was surprised that somebody could communicate with him. I felt that it was a long time since he'd had a straight conversation like this with someone. He was open to this communication, but when he saw that spirit guides and angels were surrounding him he showed fear.

I understood that since childhood, he had always seen spirits and angels from other dimensions, but he never learned how to create a filter for himself. He never knew how to recognize which ones were a positive influence and which were not. During the session I felt the urge to explain to him how he can figure out the difference. After this conversation he seemed to be more calm and receptive.

I helped him to have more clarity in his mind and in his emotions. The session was full of love, the love that he was asking to receive. This session confirmed to me that some people labeled as schizophrenic, could very well be sensitive people that don't know how to manage their sensitivity. They hear or see something that "regular people" cannot. I wonder if they received the right training at an early age, from a spiritually sensitive person, how beneficial it could be for them.

After the session Cody's mother went to visit him. He was upset but she was happy, because for the first time in a long time, he was expressing himself with thoughts and articulated sentences. When she informed me of Cody's reaction, I decided to work with him and help him to better manage his emotions. I really didn't want him to be over-medicated by the person in charge at the residential home.

I explained to him that it was perfect to show some emotions, but in a way that people didn't have a hard time dealing with him. I also explained to him how his mother and sister loved him. Indeed, they asked me to offer these sessions.

Cody's mother came back to visit him some days later, this time Cody hugged his mother and said to her: "Mom I love you!" This act was unusual for him, as Cody never wanted to be hugged or hug anybody else his entire life. His mother wrote me that this was the best gift that she had ever received from Cody.

I have been working with Cody for several months now. He seems to be very cooperative and open. I don't know where Cody will take us, but he is more balanced and calm, and he is starting to use less medication. The fact that he is having a better connection with his family is a big milestone.

In Italy I have had different cases of teen-agers who lack self esteem, are cut off spiritually, or were under too much environmental pressure, and I helped them to finally get back to their paths. I don't fix them, I only help them to clear their minds and hearts.

Such was the case with Francesco. His parents were from Italy, and they asked me to help their son. He was hav-ing a hard time deciding about his future. He had finished his degree, and he wasn't sure if he wanted to go to the university.

After my distance work with him, Francesco's mother wrote me that Francesco appeared more serene, and he had decided to go to work instead of the university. He started working in a greengrocer, and he was happy. His mother said that Francesco was very connected to nature and she felt that this was her son's way of finding this connection. They preferred to have a happy and serene son, rather than one that was stressed and unhappy.

Rita from Mexico, was having a very "dark period" in her young life. She was fifteen, and her mother was very concerned about her. She was very emotional at school, and before any test she would become ill, having to run to the restroom and throw up. She was very anxious and she was ADD. She was having strong headaches and was becoming very introverted. She wore dark clothes and preferred to stay in front of the computer as often as she could. Rita's mother was also concerned because her daughter had started to date a boy who treated her abusively.

During the first distance session, I noticed that Rita was having a hard time finding a role model as a woman. She was confused and she told me that she wanted to punish herself because she wasn't doing anything to help her mother. In some way, she felt guilty that she had been witness to her mother having been "under her father's thumb." Rita explained to me that she was upset with her mother, because she didn't stand up to her husband, Rita's father.

Consuelo Cassotti B.S.

Rita was sixteen, and she was having a hard time accepting the idea of seeing her mother treated like a "doormat."

During the session I explained to Rita that everybody has a path, a lesson to learn. I also told her that though it was painful, she needed to accept her mother's choice.

After Rita's session, I discussed with Rita's mother what her daughter was feeling, and she decided to have a session too. It was nice to see that during her session, Rita's mother was beginning to wake up and remember her beauty as a soul and woman.

After some sessions with both of them, they began to talk a little more. Rita's mother found taking a more direct approach to be more effective for her and her daughter, and it enabled her to face some of her problems with her husband. Rita better understood her mother's choices, and had less emotional problems at school. She left her boyfriend for some other girls that have the same interests.

When I work with teen-agers that are addicted to computers like Rita and others, I notice that it is like clearing them of low and heavy energies. It seems like the Internet helps trash and heavy thoughts to occupy space in their minds, and disconnects them from their hearts. When I am working with these individuals in my sessions, I feel the mind goes into a loop and it is difficult for them to come out, particularly if the person suffers from any attention disorder.

Internet is important and useful, but overuse can be powerful, and can alienate young minds. It is important to control the use and the abuse of any electronic devices.

෨෨෪

I have other great success stories, from many countries. Most are of adult clients, who if there isn't a particular disease, for different reasons are looking for some help and more awareness. Distance sessions are very powerful. Sometimes, when I give a phone session, a client can describe sensations and visualizations during the entire session. Even when they cannot, they still feel the difference in the days following the session.

I also notice that after a few sessions, people become more sensitive and can feel or sense more. I think this happens because a client becomes more aware of his/her body and his/her energy.

We live in a society that doesn't teach us how to pay attention to our body, feelings, emotions, and follow that intuitive voice inside of us. The more we allow ourselves to be open to listening, the more we can be independent and stand up for what we really want and believe.

Conclusions

I will never stop emphasizing how important it is that everyone in the family pursues a self-healing program; especially in families where there is a child with autistic spectrum disorder or other special needs.

I have seen fathers ashamed and challenged by their emotions, have a really difficult time letting go of the stigma, until they decided to have a session or have counseling. I've seen needy mothers who were sub-consciously afraid to lose their babies, any time the child showed signs of becoming more independent, with the possibility of becoming more like other children.

Unless the parents worked on themselves too, any work that I did with the child stopped sooner or later, not because of the child, but because of the parents.

In my sessions I can feel, see, and hear information that is important for me to understand in order to help the child. Sometimes the child "tells" me that the parents fight and yell too much, or they are ashamed of their "abnormal" child. They may have suicidal thoughts, or may have reached some point in time where they wished that they never had a child like him/her ... It is ok!

There is no judgment in what I see. I can understand how hard it is to be in this situation everyday. These parents are challenged every minute of the day- physically, mentally, emotionally, and spiritually. The child opens his/her heart to me and the soul connects with me. He/she trusts me. I need to listen and be truthful. Honoring the person in front of me is the only way that I can do this work.

I do my best to express to the parents only that information which is necessary, but sometimes they aren't prepared to face the truth.

This is why if they work on themselves too, there is more harmony in the whole family, and they can be more open to shift with their child.

I cannot predict what is going to happen each time I give a session. Because I am open to any possibility, I surrender myself and become a "tool" for my Angels, Archangels and Spirits Guides.

Every session is different and the results are different, mostly not because of me, but because of my clients. There is no judgment in this, for everyone has his/her own timing. Sometimes a client will see results or the shift in one session, or it may take more sessions and they see the results over time. This happens for various reasons. Perhaps we are working on very deep emotions/trauma, and it takes time to release it, or the person cannot move through the process so quickly, or has a hard time facing all the emotions. Sometimes they don't completely believe in the possibility of healing, or they are afraid to open up to this work...

What I would like to explain is this: **everyone is as unique as the result.**

We are in a time of conscious evolution. This type of evolution can be instantaneous, through shifts in consciousness. Everything can take effect immediately. Personal evolution, global evolution, universal evolution...

Everyone has the opportunity to choose to be part of this, consciously. We have the choice to consciously evolve by creating the intention, and enjoying the lesson we decide to learn everyday.

The synchronicity of events and the connections in our life, demonstrate to us that we are part of something bigger; the more we become conscious of our personal evolution, the more we become part of our global evolution.

I hope that soon more families and people everywhere will realize how important it is to become more aware of our power, and conscious of the evolution that is happening at this time. When we learn to listen to our inner voice, we change the belief systems that create the cage of our life.

We are surrounded by angels and high beings, who are willing to help us every day, if we ask and listen. God/Goddess or the Source has given us free will, and our Guardian Angel and Spirits Guides will not overstep this. When we suspend our disbelief, we become open to any possibility.

Observing my clients as they become more open to listening to their intuitive voices and realizing that they are supported in their own paths, brings joy to my heart every time. Recognizing who we are and what our mission is, is an important step. The more we realize the connection, the big picture that we are part of, the more we can flow with harmony and share this possibility with others.

I am still learning from the children and people that I meet, and I am still amazed by the shifts and changes that one can make in such a short time... when ready. I feel

Consuelo Cassotti B.S.

blessed to have such deep friendships supporting me whenever I am in need, from both this reality and others.

I want to thank them all; for laughing at me and with me anytime I am too serious, or telling the truth even when I don't like to hear it. I am human and I am here to learn, like everyone else.

About the author

Consuelo Cassotti as International Teacher and Intuitive Healer travels back and forth between Italy and the United States, combining her holistic teaching activities with her holistic sessions.

Consuelo's work is a unique and intuitive combination of various methods that she uses during her classes and her sessions. She can regenerate cells, help energy shift, release emotional-trauma blocks from present life and past lives, and helps to download information necessary to be prepared for the "Big Shift".

"Energy Balancing and Awakening the Soul" session is a method that Consuelo has achieved after years of studying and experiencing. It is based on the extraction/synthesis of several holistic methods combined together.

She works in Dayton and Columbus area (OH), Chicago (IL) and North Italy. BalancEvolution, LLC.

For any information or to contact her:

www.balancEvolution.com
www.AutismSolutionsOhio.com

Made in the USA
Charleston, SC
05 May 2013